Environmental Bioethics

Environmental bioethics addresses the environmental impact of the health care industry and climate change health hazards as two ethical issues which impact each other. This edited volume examines the theory of environmental bioethics and offers practical examples of practices which make health care more sustainable.

Written in an accessible style which allows readers to understand what environmental bioethics is and why it is important, this book presents real-life case studies and thoughtful reflections from leading doctors, clinicians, and ethicists. Contributions to this volume address ethical frameworks for environmental bioethics and delve into the role of doctors in environmentally sustainable health care. Together, they offer hope for a more sustainable health care industry while also recognizing how much more needs to be done.

A key resource for scholars, practitioners, and researchers of philosophy, environmental studies, public health, and the allied health sciences, this book will also be relevant to international policymakers, especially in countries which have socialized health care (such as those in the EU), who want a rationale for health care decarbonization and practical examples. It will also appeal to educated citizens, particularly those who demand positive environmental change and are interested in the concept of sustainable health care. This book was originally published as a special issue of *The New Bioethics*.

Cristina Richie, PhD, is Lecturer in Ethics of Technology at the Centre for Technomoral Futures at the University of Edinburgh, UK, and one of the leading global ethicists in sustainable health care. In addition to being Joint Editor of *Global Bioethics*, Dr Richie is the author of two monographs and over fifty articles.

Environmental Bioethics

Theory and Practice for Environmentally Sustainable Health Care

Edited by
Cristina Richie

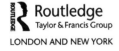

LONDON AND NEW YORK

First published 2024
by Routledge
4 Park Square, Milton Park, Abingdon, Oxon, OX14 4RN

and by Routledge
605 Third Avenue, New York, NY 10158

Routledge is an imprint of the Taylor & Francis Group, an informa business
© 2024 Taylor & Francis

All rights reserved. No part of this book may be reprinted or reproduced or utilised in any form or by any electronic, mechanical, or other means, now known or hereafter invented, including photocopying and recording, or in any information storage or retrieval system, without permission in writing from the publishers.

Trademark notice: Product or corporate names may be trademarks or registered trademarks, and are used only for identification and explanation without intent to infringe.

British Library Cataloguing-in-Publication Data
A catalogue record for this book is available from the British Library

ISBN13: 978-1-032-73729-4 (hbk)
ISBN13: 978-1-032-73730-0 (pbk)
ISBN13: 978-1-003-46565-2 (ebk)

DOI: 10.4324/9781003465652

Typeset in Minion Pro
by codeMantra

Publisher's Note
The publisher accepts responsibility for any inconsistencies that may have arisen during the conversion of this book from journal articles to book chapters, namely the inclusion of journal terminology.

Disclaimer
Every effort has been made to contact copyright holders for their permission to reprint material in this book. The publishers would be grateful to hear from any copyright holder who is not here acknowledged and will undertake to rectify any errors or omissions in future editions of this book.

Contents

Citation Information vii
Notes on Contributors ix

Foreword: Nature Bites Back 1
Trevor Stammers

Introduction – Sustainability and Bioethics: Where We Have Been, Where
We Are, Where We Are Going 2
Cristina Richie

PART I
Ethical Theory for Environmental Bioethics 11

1 Does Health Promotion Harm the Environment? 13
   Cheryl C. Macpherson, Elise Smith and Travis N. Rieder

2 Bioethics and Environmental Ethics: The Story of the Human Body as a
   Natural Ecosystem 31
   Zoe-Athena Papalois and Kyriaki-Barbara Papalois

3 Restorative Commons as an Expanded Ethical Framework for Public Health
   and Environmental Sustainability 38
   Robert Gurevich

PART II
Ethical Practice for Environmentally Sustainable Health Care 53

4 The Climate Emergency: Are the Doctors who take Non-violent Direct
   Action to Raise Public Awareness Radical Activists, Rightminded
   Professionals, or Reluctant Whistleblowers? 55
   Terry Kemple

5 Will the Plant-Based movement Redefine Physicians' Understanding of
   Chronic Disease? 69
   Maximilian Andreas Storz

6   Going Green: Decreasing Medical Waste in a Paediatric Intensive Care Unit
    in the United States   86
    Zelda J. Ghersin, Michael R. Flaherty, Phoebe Yager and Brian M. Cummings

Index   99

Citation Information

The chapters in this book were originally published in the journal *The New Bioethics*, volume 26, issue 2 (2020). When citing this material, please use the original page numbering for each article, as follows:

Foreword
   Nature bites back
   Trevor Stammers
   The New Bioethics, volume 26, issue 2 (2020) pp. 81

Introduction
   Guest Editorial: Sustainability and bioethics: where we have been, where we are, where we are going
   Cristina Richie
   The New Bioethics, volume 26, issue 2 (2020) pp. 82–90

Chapter 1
   Does Health Promotion Harm the Environment?
   Cheryl C. Macpherson, Elise Smith and Travis N. Rieder
   The New Bioethics, volume 26, issue 2 (2020) pp. 158–175

Chapter 2
   Bioethics and Environmental Ethics: The Story of the Human Body as a Natural Ecosystem
   Zoe-Athena Papalois and Kyriaki-Barbara Papalois
   The New Bioethics, volume 26, issue 2 (2020) pp. 91–97

Chapter 3
   Restorative Commons as an Expanded Ethical Framework for Public Health and Environmental Sustainability
   Robert Gurevich
   The New Bioethics, volume 26, issue 2 (2020) pp. 125–140

Chapter 4
   The Climate Emergency: Are the Doctors who take Non-violent Direct Action to Raise Public Awareness Radical Activists, Rightminded Professionals, or Reluctant Whistleblowers?
   Terry Kemple
   The New Bioethics, volume 26, issue 2 (2020) pp. 111–124

Chapter 5
Will the Plant-Based movement Redefine Physicians' Understanding of Chronic Disease?
Maximilian Andreas Storz
The New Bioethics, volume 26, issue 2 (2020) pp. 141–157

Chapter 6
Going Green: Decreasing Medical Waste in a Paediatric Intensive Care Unit in the United States
Zelda J. Ghersin, Michael R. Flaherty, Phoebe Yager and Brian M. Cummings
The New Bioethics, volume 26, issue 2 (2020) pp. 98–110

For any permission-related enquiries please visit:
http://www.tandfonline.com/page/help/permissions

Notes on Contributors

Brian M. Cummings is a pediatric intensivist, as well as Medical Director and Vice Chair for the Department of Pediatrics at Massachusetts General Hospital, and Executive Director for the Clinical Process Improvement Leadership Program (CPIP) at Mass General Brigham.

Michael R. Flaherty is Director for Pediatric Inpatient Quality and Safety at Massachusetts General Hospital for Children and an instructor in Pediatrics at Harvard Medical School, Boston, USA.

Zelda J. Ghersin is a board-certified pediatric intensivist who specializes in the care of critically ill children and infants. She completed her fellowship training at Massachusetts General Hospital and Harvard Medical School, Boston, USA.

Robert Gurevich is Chief Financial Officer at Brooklyn Free Clinic at SUNY Downstate College of Medicine, USA. His interest in sustainability began in Brooklyn College, where he majored in Business for Health Professions, following an urban ecology project that involved tracking coyote migrations through green corridors in NYC.

Terry Kemple was a full time GP in Bristol for 30 years until his retirement. He has had roles in teaching, research, management, and quality improvement. He was President of the RCGP 2015-2017 and since 2017 its national representative for Sustainability, Climate Change and Green issues.

Cheryl C. Macpherson is Professor and Chair of the Bioethics Department in the School of Medicine at St. George's University (SGU), Grenada. Her research interests include environmental and public health ethics.

Zoe-Athena Papalois is a fourth year medical student at King's College London, iBSc Human Anatomy and Developmental Biology, IME member, and ASGBI medical student apprentice.

Kyriaki-Barbara Papalois is an academic foundation doctor at the Royal Berkshire NHS Foundation Trust, UK.

Cristina Richie, PhD, is Lecturer in Ethics of Technology at the Centre for Technomoral Futures at the University of Edinburgh, UK, and one of the leading global ethicists in sustainable health care. In addition to being Joint Editor of *Global Bioethics*, Dr Richie is the author of two monographs and over fifty articles.

Travis N. Rieder is Assistant Director for Education Initiatives, Director of the Master of Bioethics degree program, and Research Scholar at the Berman Institute of Bioethics. His interests include ethics and policy questions about sustainability and planetary limits and responsible procreation in the era of climate change.

Elise Smith is Assistant Professor in the Department of Preventive Medicine and Population Health (PMPH) at the University of Texas Medical Branch, Galveston, USA. With a background in philosophy, law, and the social sciences, she works on projects in research ethics, research integrity, and public health ethics.

Trevor Stammers is Honorary Senior Research Fellow at Spurgeons College, UK. He served as the editor of the journal *The New Bioethics* from 20011 to 2023. His recent publication includes *The Ethics of Global Organ Acquisition: Moral Arguments about Transplantation*.

Maximilian Andreas Storz is a medical doctor from Germany. His main interests include plant-based whole-food diets and lifestyle medicine. He is also interested in climate change, animal welfare, and environmental sustainability.

Phoebe Yager is Chief of Pediatric Critical Care Medicine at Massachusetts General Hospital for Children. She is a pediatric intensivist, specializing in the care of critically ill and injured infants, children, and adolescents.

Foreword: Nature bites back

This themed edition on environmental ethics was commissioned a long time before reports first began to emerge from China about an epidemic of a previously unknown viral infection. By the summer of 2020, the whole world is grappling with the devastation that the Covid-19 disease complex is still wreaking at the time of publication now, let alone the death toll and economic collapse it has already left in its first wave. Covid-19 and environmental exploitation are two major global threats. Covid-19 has been taken seriously because it kills quickly; climate change is still being ignored by many but may yet kill far greater numbers.

I am then more indebted than usual to our guest editor, Prof Cristina Richie, for bringing together this fascinating and yet troubling collection of papers, which I hope will help increase awareness of how important health care is in raising the profile of climate change on the bioethical agenda. In my first decade of being Editor in Chief, I have never known an edition to come together under such pressure and yet with such determination. I hope it will provoke change in actions as well as in the thinking of our readers. Who knows where we will be with either Covid or climate trends by the next issue? Whatever, this edition contributes to making both situations that little bit less dangerous.

ORCID

Trevor Stammers http://orcid.org/0000-0002-4454-2501

Trevor Stammers
Editor In Chief
trevor.stammers@stmarys.ac.uk

Introduction – Sustainability and Bioethics: Where We Have Been, Where We Are, Where We Are Going

CRISTINA RICHIE

Where we have been

Bioethics, as we are too infrequently reminded, was originally an ethical system concerned with the 'problems of interference with other living beings ... and generally everything related to the balance of the ecosystem' according to the 1978 Encyclopedia of Bioethics (Reich 1978). This definition was predicated on the work of two men – Frtiz Jahr in Germany – and Van Rensselaer Potter in the United States.

In 1927, German minister Fritz Jahr described bio-ethics (German: *bio-ethik*) as 'the assumption of moral obligations not only towards humans, but towards all forms of life' (Jahr and Sass 2010). Jahr drew on Rudolf Eisler's *Bio-Psychik*, which was 'the science of the soul of all, what lives' to underpin his philosophy of bio-ethics and ultimately promoted a Western, deontological articulation of bioethics, rather than an Eastern, consequentialist bioethic. Jahr summarizes his philosophy by declaring, 'Respect every living being on principle as an end in itself and treat it, if possible, as such!' Almost half a century later, the term 'bioethics' appeared in English.

In 1971, Van Rensselaer Potter advanced the term bioethic as a way to describe 'a global perspective with an ecological focus on how we as humans will guide our adaptations to our environment' (Potter 1971). This life (*bios*) ethic emerged from a tangible need to evaluate the actions of humans in an industrialized society struggling within a precarious ecosystem. Trained as an oncologist, Potter was particularly sensitive to the connections between health and habitat. Thus, he conceptualized a humanistic ethical system rooted in an intrinsically practical approach to sustainable life, inclusive of the earth and other organisms (Potter 1988). The *bios* in bioethics is inextricably connected to conservation and medicine.

The ethical commitments of bioethics were initially much more robust than the four principles of biomedical ethics. Conceptually, bioethics was also much broader than the patient-physician relationship. The scope was global, not local; inclusive, not exclusive. And while the development of bioethics as an academic discipline – which was formerly attentive to nature and ecosystems – into a more technological-individual field gave the appearance that ecology is separate from medicine, there have always been scholars and literature where the twain meet. This juncture is most commonly referred to as environmental bioethics.

As an interdisciplinary field, the breadth of biomedical topics which have been folded into environmental bioethics – or addressed with an environmental ethos – are striking. Environmental bioethics, as an applied discipline, takes shape through initiatives in many parts of the world. The United Kingdom's National Health Services (NHS) and the United States' Catholic Health Association have emerged as organizational leaders in environmental bioethics in recent decades.

Significantly, the UK is the only region of the world that integrates sustainable health care policy into their national health system. The UK's model of environmental bioethics relies on legal standards to enforce carbon reduction measures in the NHS. Following from the United Kingdom Climate Change Act of 2008 (UK Public General Acts 2008), the document *Saving Carbon, Improving Health: NHS Carbon Reduction Strategy for England* encouraged carbon-neutral transportation – like walking and biking – eliminating animal-based foods from menus, and reducing water waste in health care facilities (National Health Services Sustainable Development Unit 2009). A complementary document from the National Institutes for Health Research, 'highlights areas where sensible research design can reduce waste without adversely impacting the validity and reliability of research' 2010). Similarly, the NHS *Climate Change Strategy for Wales* released in 2010 (National Health Services 2010), outlined policies for sustainable health care based on the groundbreaking data from the *Carbon Footprint of NHS Wales 2005–2009* study (Lungley 2010). As a comprehensive system of sustainable health care in the UK, efforts in Scotland to reduce carbon emissions include NHS Scotland's *Climate Change Plan* (National Health Services Health Scotland 2017) and support from the Scottish Public Health Network and Scottish Managed Sustainable Health Network (SMASH), which also addresses climate change health hazards (Conacher 2019).

The UK model of environmental bioethics depends on the carbon calculations of health care. In addition to the rather straightforward carbon calculations of health care buildings, increasingly studies are published on the carbon emissions of individual medical procedures. Data is available on cataract operations (Morris *et al.* 2013), heart bypass operations (Berners-Lee 2010), conventional hemodialysis (Lim *et al.* 2013), caesarian sections and vaginal childbirth (Campion *et al.* 2012), hysterectomies (Woods *et al.* 2013), Critical Care Unit stays (Pollard *et al.* 2014), randomized controlled trials (Lyle *et al.* 2009), and a variety of dental services (Duane *et al.* 2017). Carbon calculations are a valuable tool in determining the environmental impact of health care, while also meeting the desires that many patients, practitioners, and health care facilities have to understand the impact of their health choices on the environment.

The NHS continues to systematically address methods for minimizing the carbon impact of health care. Current initiatives include a commitment to reduce single use plastics (Courtney-Guy 2019) and decrease the use of certain anesthetic gasses (Bawden 2019). A thorough evaluation of 'social prescribing' of pharmaceuticals is significant, since prescription drugs are the second largest contributor to health care carbon emissions in the NHS, after medical instruments and equipment (Sustainable Development Unit 2018). Recently, the Newcastle upon Tyne Hospitals NHS Foundation Trust declared a climate emergency, which several other NHS Foundations Trusts have endorsed (Wise 2020). These actions, in addition to education about sustainable health care in medical school curriculum (Walpole *et al.* 2015, Maxwell and Blashki 2016, Walpole and Mortimer 2017), provide a clear and consistent response to the environmental impact of health care.

In contrast to the UK, the US has a decentralized approach to sustainable health care, which codifies environmental ethics into hospitals and health care policy, supported by the oversight of organizations. Health Care Without Harm, Practice Greenhealth, and the Healthier Hospitals Initiative offer umbrella programmes for individual health care facilities to join voluntarily. However, the Catholic Health Association (CHA) with 'more than 600 hospitals and 1,600 long-term care and other health facilities in all 50 states is the largest group of nonprofit health care providers in the nation'. The CHA creates and implements their own environmental initiatives, which, given their size, is significant in environmental bioethics.

Employees at many CHA hospitals are educated about environmental health and encouraged to recycle paper, carpool, reduce waste in the workplace, and support renewable forms of energy (Florida Medical Association 2015). Health care facilities endorse sustainable design, energy conservation, waste reduction, minimizing bottled water, and eliminating mercury-containing devices. The Catholic Health Association has gone beyond organizational models of sustainable health care by engaging communities in gardening and lobbying for better government support for the environment.

Catholic Health Association initiatives are undeniably tied to Catholic identity and are 'woven into the very fabric of Catholic mission' (Catholic Health Association and Practice Greenhealth 2010). As an organization that advocates a 'seamless garment' of respect for all life, the CHA simultaneously works for eco-justice and social justice, noting that the two are connected. In 2020, Pope Francis recognized that 'a true ecological approach always becomes a social approach; it must integrate questions of justice in debates on the environment, so as to hear both the cry of the earth and the cry of the poor' (Pope Francis 2020). By drawing on common values that cross denominational lines – such as health and stewardship – the CHA is able to provide optimal patient care while also maintaining rigorous environmental standards.

Environmental bioethics, which at once addresses the environmental impact of the medical industry (Pichler *et al.* 2019), and climate change health hazards, is a dynamic discipline. Simultaneously, thematic elements such as interconnectedness of planetary health and human health, dedication to living in harmony with nature – of which humans are part – and emphasis on systems and symbiosis remains unchanged. This issue of *The New Bioethics* is not only a celebration of nearly a century of environmental bioethics, but also a reiteration of its necessity today.

Where we are

The original concept of bioethics – both in English speaking and non-English speaking milieus – was attentive to biotic life around us, indicating that environmental aspects of health and obligations to care for each other and our environment were core commitments. Even so, the intellectual starting point of environmental bioethics is significantly different than biomedical ethics. Instead of thinking of technology, medical intervention, and the individual first, environmental bioethics takes an almost primordial approach to health and upends the modern ideology that humans and nature are dissimilar. Zoe-Athena Papalois and Kyriaki-Barbara Papalois' lead article does double duty in this respect (Papalois and Papalois 2020). It first, acts as a wake up call to those slumbering in the artificially crafted world of technology. It second, draws rich and complicated parallels between the human body and the planet. The examples offered in 'Bioethics and Environmental Ethics: The Story of the Human Body as a Natural Ecosystem' are more than analogical; they are parallel descriptors of an intricate system of life that exists in a coherent matrix. To quote the authors, homeostasis 'describes the human body's intrinsic tendency towards equilibrium. A change in one direction elicits a response in the opposite direction, restoring harmony. An excessive shift results in a change that cannot be compensated. This imbalance results in illness'. Much like the body, the environment also strives for equilibrium. Significantly, the Papalois' offer an ecological paradigm to a medical community who primarily conceptualize illness in terms of physical function. By demonstrating that the earth is also a system, which can be well or sick, health care professionals can begin to understand the methodological approach – and contribution of – environmental bioethics. Indeed, some health care professionals are already leading the way.

Four doctors based at the Harvard Medical School-affiliated Massachusetts General Hospital (MGH) for Children detail their initiatives to reduce waste in a pediatric intensive care unit (PICU). Zelda J. Ghersin, Brian M. Cummings, Michael Flaherty, and Phoebe Yager evaluate the medical resources used and disposed of when our bodies become sick (Ghersin *et al.* 2020). In the PICU, as well as NICUs and ICUs, an enormous amount of hospital waste is generated. While hospital policies on 'medical waste' are appropriately based on safety standards, there is little reflection about alternatives which maintain sterility and reduce the carbon footprint of health care. The authors note that medical personnel 'must find ways to balance the professional duty to prepare with the professional duty to limit the negative impact practices have on the environment, and to save resources when able.' Hence, the 'Green Team' at MGH emerged as a task force which calculated, and thereby tangibly reduced, the amount of medical waste produced in the course of patient care. Their successful endeavour is detailed in 'Going Greener:

Decreasing Medical Waste in a Pediatric Intensive Care Unit' and is one of only a handful of published quantifiable studies on medical waste in hospitals.

Much like the US-based doctors, UK physician Terry Kemple underscores the tension between professional obligations to protect patients from harm and the impending health threats from climate change (Kemple 2020). Kemple draws upon ethical theories and medical codes to demonstrate that physicians are accountable for patient and public health. Recipients of medical care must be given the best care, not only at the moment of need, but also in the long-run. Medical organizations, such as the General Medical Council, endorse this duty by 'providing a comprehensive overview of the obligations and professional behaviour of a doctor to their patients and wider society'. Yet, when physicians participate in non-violent actions like those organized by Extinction Rebellion (XR), they may be censured. Arrests of doctor-activists can lead to a GMC tribunal, despite the apparent imperative to actively protect human health. 'The Climate Emergency: Are the Doctors Who Take Non-Violent Direct Action to Raise Public Awareness Radical Activists, Rightminded Professionals, or Reluctant Whistle-Blowers?' exposes the internal contradiction of some health care organizations and reinterprets traditional medical codes of conduct to not only include – but also mandate – climate action as a matter of personal integrity.

The Ghersin *et al.* and Kemple articles describe actions and initiatives that health care providers can take to minimize harm within and outside of the hospital, respectively. A complementary narrative for sustainable health care comes from environmental ethics. In 'Restorative Commons as an Expanded Ethical Framework for Public Health and Environmental Sustainability', Robert Gurevich offers a bridge between health care and ecology by providing a model of proactive sustainability (Gurevich 2020). He observes, 'current sustainability initiatives are limited in their scope; for example, targeted campaigns to reduce carbon footprints may achieve some measure of success, but they do not change humanity's relationship with the environment, which is the root of the issue'. Therefore, in recognition that humans are part of the Commons, harmonious recommendations for health are offered within and beyond the clinic. Gurevich explores the benefits of 'ecotherapy', which immerse individuals with mental and physical health conditions in nature, and green health centres, which integrate conservationist practices into the daily life of a hospital. This 'both-and' philosophy restores humans to an ecological nexus which at once protects from disease and contributes to cure. Indeed, if nature is the cure, then health care providers must be persuaded as such through scientific analysis of evidenced based medicine.

Echoing the theme of planetary and corporeal health that was highlighted in Papalois and Papalois's article, medical doctor Maximilian Andreas Storz draws parallels between the increase in global chronic disease burden and excessive carbon emissions (Storz 2020). The contemporary, Western attitude to both illness and environmental exploitation utilize a reactive model that manages the symptoms but not the disease. Questioning the conventional practice, which permits destructive habits and then offers high tech solutions, 'Will the Plant-Based Movement Redefine Physicians' Understanding of Chronic Disease?' provides indubitable evidence that vegetarian and vegan diets are not only effective in reducing and preventing disease, but also are more environmentally sustainable, as they require fewer natural resources and expend less carbon. Significantly, Storz goes beyond merely describing the benefits of eating lower on the food chain and declares, 'plant-based diets are a powerful tool – not using and advocating for them is not only unethical, but harms patients and the planet alike'. The ethical demands on health care professionals include accountability to patients and obligations to professionalism. Environmentally aware clinicians braid these two commitments into a variety of ecologically sound health care practices.

To be sure, health care providers are not the only stakeholders in sustainable medicine. The final article offers a rousing call to action for medical researchers, scientists, bioethicists, policymakers, and other individuals who must actively participate in delivering medical care that does not result in a Sisyphean cycle of pollute-treat-pollute. Cheryl Macpherson, Elise Smith, and Travis Rieder maintain, 'given the goals of healthcare, claims of and calls for health promotion are hypocritical unless they involve strategies and policies that explicitly protect environments and natural resources' (Macpherson *et al.* 2020). Health care cannot continue its current trajectory of environmental exploitation – given the widely established facts about climate change health hazards, medical resource consumption, and medical waste. Three concrete solutions are thus offered in 'Does Health Promotion Harm the Environment?': slowing the global birthrate, transforming the food system, and genetically modifying mosquitoes. Utilizing the ingenuity of science to safeguard human health and protect the planet is emphasized, demonstrating that environmental bioethics encompasses many outlooks. And still, the double-dividend approach, which works towards the common goals of satisfying the ethical standards of human rights to health and the moral imperative for environmental conservation, is the common theme in this issue of *The New Bioethics*.

Where we are going

Sustainable medicine will continue to address the most pertinent aspects of environmental health while compounding the irrefutable evidence that the health care industry must embark on a radically different path than the one it is on now. The Coronavirus pandemic highlighted the importance of environmental bioethics for health in a variety of ways. First, simply examining the biological spread of COVID-19 and the precautionary measures of social isolation and self-quarantine remind the human collective that we are all interconnected. One person's actions effect another and may set off a chain reaction that has local, national, and international implications. Although much ecological destruction is invisible to the general public, each purchase that is made, each health care procedure used, and every medical choice has an environmental impact. Humans have had to adapt to thinking in terms of long-range cause and effect by imagining the spread of Coronavirus on surfaces. An infected person may touch a product, which will be shipped to a store, which will be stocked by a worker, which will be purchased, brought home, and shared with family, thus transmitting this highly contagious virus. Humans also need to understand the carbon impact of consumerism in the same way. The creation of a product had a carbon footprint, as did the fuel used for transportation, the cooling system used in the grocery store, the emissions from the car ride home, and the disposal of the bottle. Although the immediate consequence of the resource use is unrecognized, the environmental outcome will surely be accounted for later.

Second, many people are now living in a world where movements and actions are considerably limited. There are mandated home quarantines for those of advanced age and people who are symptomatic. Road closures, domestic bans, and closed borders prevent travel. Daily updates about increased restrictions offer little warning before implementation and in some parts of the country, are not readily disseminated. Yet, these measures will become more commonplace unless carbon emissions are reduced and climate change health hazards are minimized. All adults and children will need to shelter in place when air quality compromises respiratory health. Severe weather, including hurricanes, tornados, floods, and blizzards will close access points, leaving hundreds or thousands of people stranded. As with the Coronavirus, the elderly, disabled, poor, homeless, and those with young children will be most affected.

Third, the devastating economic effects of the Coronavirus have illuminated the need to re-think commerce. Certain businesses that provide 'fast fashion', lifestyle trends, other 'non-essential' services have been curtailed, while sanitation, health care, and education are preserved. Disposable life cannot be sustained. As policymakers work towards economic recovery, more should be done to support the triple bottom line of people, planet, and profit. This includes green collar jobs with a variety of entry level positions, a green gig economy, and investment into technologies that both clean and preserve the environment.

Despite the devastating parallels between COVID-19 and climate change, the global emergency has offered windows of hope. Communities are able to discern the essential – health, family, food – from the trivial. Worldwide, people are placing emphasis on generous relationships, outdoor activity, and a marked reduction in eating and drinking out. Health care is being prioritized as a national interest, as is the necessity of keeping open spaces, such as hiking trails, parks, and sidewalks, available and well maintained. This reorientation towards low carbon activities will perhaps remind many about the emotional and spiritual goods that cannot be bought.

A prescient Van Rensselaer Potter wrote in 1971 that 'technological decisions should not be made on the basis of profit alone, but should be examined in terms of survival'. Whether in the medical industry or designing a better world, survival, here, does not mean a reckless exploitation of resources and energy. Rather, survival is dependent on the cohesion of the natural and built environment. The way back is also the way forward.

References

Bawden, A. 2019. The NHS produces 5.4% of the UK's greenhouse gases. How can hospitals cut their emissions? *The Guardian*, 18 September.

Berners-Lee, M., 2010. *How bad are bananas? The carbon footprint of everything*. London: Profile Book.

Campion, N., et al., 2012. Life cycle assessment perspectives on delivering an infant in the US. *Science of the Total Environment*, 425, 191–198.

Catholic Health Association and Practice Greenhealth, 2010. *Environmental sustainability: Getting started guide*. St. Louis: The Catholic Health Association of the United States.

Conacher, A., 2019. SMaSH Workplan: To be read in conjunction with the Work Programme 2017-20 Work Plan Activity 2019-20. *Scottish Managed Sustainable Health Network*, 1–5.

Courtney-Guy, S. 2019. NHS vows to cut single-use plastic by up to half. *Metro*, 12 October.

Duane, B., et al., 2017. An estimated carbon footprint of NHS primary dental care within England. How can dentistry be more environmentally sustainable? *British Dental Journal*, 223, 589–593.

Florida Medical Association and My Green Doctor. 2015. Workbook 2: Renewable Energy. Available from: http://www.mygreendoctor.org/workbook-2-introduction/ [Accessed 8 April, 2020].

Ghersin, Z., et al., 2020. Going greener: Decreasing medical waste in a pediatric intensive care unit. *The New Bioethics*, 26 (2).

Gurevich, R., 2020. Restorative commons as an expanded ethical framework for public health and environmental sustainability. *The New Bioethics*, 26 (2).

Jahr, F., and Sass, H.-M., 2010. Bio—ethics—reviewing the ethical relations of humans towards animals and plants. *JAHR-European Journal of Bioethics*, 1, 227–231.

Kemple, T., 2020. The climate emergency: Are the doctors who take non-violent direct action to raise public awareness radical Activists, rightminded professionals, or reluctant whistle-blowers? *The New Bioethics*, 26 (2).

Lim, A.E., et al., 2013. The carbon footprint of an Australian satellite haemodialysis unit. *Australian Health Review*, 37, 369–74.

Lungley, H., 2010. *Carbon Footprint of NHS Wales 2005-2009*. New York: GHD.

Lyle, K., et al., 2009. Carbon cost of pragmatic randomised controlled trials: retrospective analysis of sample of trials. *BMJ*, 339, b4187.

Macpherson, C., et al., 2020. Does health promotion harm the environment? *The New Bioethics*, 26 (2).

Maxwell, J. and Blashki, G., 2016. Teaching about climate change in medical education: an opportunity. *Journal of Public Health Research*, 5 (673), 14–20.

Morris, D.S., et al., 2013. The carbon footprint of cataract surgery. *Eye*, 27, 495–501.

National Health Services, 2010. *Climate change strategy for Wales summary*. Version Crown.

National Health Services Health Scotland, 2017. *A Fairer Healthier Scotland -A strategic framework for action 2017-2022*. Edinburgh: NHS Health Scotland.

National Health Services Sustainable Development Unit, 2009. *Saving carbon, improving health: NHS carbon reduction strategy for England*. London: NHS Sustainable Development Unit.

National Institutes for Health Research. 2010. Carbon Reduction Guidelines. October.

Papalois, Z.-A. and Papalois, K.-B., 2020. Bioethics and Environmental Ethics: The Story of the Human Body as a Natural Ecosystem. *The New Bioethics*, 26 (2).

Pichler, P.-P., et al., 2019. International comparison of health care carbon footprints. *Environmental Research Letters*, 14, 064004.

Pollard, A.S., et al., 2014. The carbon footprint of acute care: how energy intensive is critical care? *Public health*, 128, 771–776.

Pope Francis, 2020. Querida Amazonia. Esortazione Apostolica post-sinodale, 12 February. Available from: https://press.vatican.va/content/salastampa/it/bollettino/pubblico/2020/02/12/0091/00189.html#ing [Acessed 8 April, 2020].

Potter, V.R., 1971. *Bioethics: Bridge to the future*. Upper Saddle River, NJ: Prentice-Hall.

———., 1988. *Global bioethics: Building on the leopold legacy*. East Lansing, MI: Michigan State University Press.

Reich, W.T., ed. 1978. *The Encyclopedia of bioethics, vol. 1*. New York: Macmillan.

Storz, M.A., 2020. Will the plant-based movement redefine physicians' understanding of chronic disease? *The New Bioethics*, 26 (2).

Sustainable Development Unit for NHS England and Public Health England. 2018. Reducing the Use of natural resources in health and social care.

UK Public General Acts. 2008. Climate Change Act.

Walpole, S.C., *et al.*, 2015. Exploring emerging learning needs: a UK-wide consultation on environmental sustainability learning objectives for medical education. *International journal of medical education*, 6, 191–200.

Walpole, S.C., and Mortimer, F., 2017. Evaluation of a collaborative project to develop sustainable healthcare education in eight UK medical schools. *Public health*, 150, 134–148.

Wise, J., 2020. Climate emergency: new expert panel will set out how NHS can achieve net zero. *BMJ*, 368, m310–m310.

Woods, D., *et al.*, 2013. Comparison of the environmental impact of commonly used surgical approaches to hysterectomy. *Gynecologic Oncology*, 130, e143–e143.

Part I
Ethical Theory for Environmental Bioethics

Does Health Promotion Harm the Environment?

CHERYL C. MACPHERSON

ELISE SMITH

TRAVIS N. RIEDER

Health promotion involves social and environmental interventions designed to benefit and protect health. It often harmfully impacts the environment through air and water pollution, medical waste, greenhouse gas emissions, and other externalities. We consider potential conflicts between health promotion and environmental protection and why and how the healthcare industry might promote health while protecting environments. After probing conflicts between promoting health and protecting the environment we highlight the essential role that environmental resources play in health and healthcare to show that environmental protection is a form of health promotion. We then explore relationships between three radical forms of health promotion and the environment: (1) lowering the human birth rate; (2) transforming the food system; and (3) genetically modifying mosquitos. We conclude that healthcare and other industries and their institutions and leaders have responsibilities to re-consider and modify their priorities, policies, and practices.

Introduction

Health promotion involves 'a wide range of social and environmental interventions that are designed to benefit and protect individual people's health and quality of life by addressing and preventing the root causes of ill health, not just focusing on treatment and cure' (World Health Organization 2016). Health promotion is conducted in medical, nursing, dental, public health, and other realms of healthcare. It is consistent with collaborative, transdisciplinary, and multisectoral approaches such as 'One Health' – a field which aims to benefit human and animal health by documenting and conceptualizing disease processes linking people, animals, and the environment (Centers for Disease Control 2019). Evidence supporting these interconnections comes from many fields. Examples include clinical epidemiology which documents how specific determinants of health are linked to various environmental factors; molecular biology which examines, among others, environmental impacts on gene expression (Dupras *et al.* 2014); and public health which explores interconnected models and influences of antimicrobial resistance and industrial pollution on humans and nature (Land and Rayner 2012). Examining the need for environmental protection of wildlife, marine life, plants, water sources and clean air is the *raison d'être* for many fields of study including environmental ethics and environmental sciences.

Environments and the natural resources they encompass and connect with are essential to human health and wellbeing. Bioethics, in its earliest years, was concerned with interdisciplinary dialogue about relationships between human individuals and populations; the natural and socio-political environments in which they exist and with which they interact; and the natural resources on which health and wellbeing depend (Potter 1971). Contemporary bioethics is more anthropocentric, values human health above all else, and tends to address environmental protections secondarily or leaves them out altogether. Few publications or debates in contemporary bioethics acknowledge environmental considerations but bioethics journals and conferences are increasingly turning toward ethical questions about interconnections between human health, healthcare, and environments (Macpherson 2013, Macpherson 2014).

When health promotion policies and practices conflict with environmental policies and practices there are consequences for human health. Regulatory controls that protect against air or water pollution involve practical and ethical considerations about their efficacy, the harms likely to occur in their absence, and the value of promoting and prioritizing human health over at least some activities of industrial polluters. Ethical values of decisionmakers and regulatory bodies influence the extent to which controls, policies, and practices are grounded in empirical evidence, enacted, and upheld and this has health consequences because relationships exist between health promotion, environments, and environmental resources for health such as clean air and water (Jamieson 2014).

The influence of the numerous institutions, organizations, and activities that promote health increases the complexity of healthcare and its delivery and sometimes confounds decision-making and implementation. Collectively, these bodies and their components comprise the 'medical industrial complex' or 'healthcare industry' (Relman 1980). Globally, the healthcare industry today contributes an abundance of diagnostic tests and treatments that are widely used and overused, create unnecessary waste, damage environments and environmental resources, and create need for environmental protections; this puts at least some goals of health promotion in conflict with goals of environmental protection (Resnik 2009). Environmental impacts of health promotion differ in prevalence and severity and are often harmful. They include the steadily rising burden of greenhouse gas emissions and climate change with many empirically documented and measured health and environmental impacts.

We explore conflicts between health promotion and environmental protection and highlight associated ethical considerations and responsibilities across the healthcare industry. After contextualizing the conflicting goals to show that health promotion does indeed harm environments, we argue that this creates a responsibility within the healthcare industry and its institutions to protect environments by adopting environmentally friendly policies and practices that do not compromise access to, or standards of, healthcare. We discuss three radical health promotion projects and their environmental impacts: (1) lowering the global human birth rate in order to provide healthcare to present and future people around the world; (2) transforming food systems from production through consumption and waste disposal in order to protect Earth's capacity to nourish and feed its global population (by 2050, global population is projected to reach 10 billion and outweigh Earth's capacity to sustainably provide healthy food for all); and (3) genetically modifying mosquitos to reduce human exposure to and infection with mosquito-borne diseases.

Relationships between health promotion and the environment

The perspectives of contemporary bioethics and environmental ethics differ but connect through Van Rensselaer Potter's construct of bioethics as an interdisciplinary field concerned with relationships between health and environments (Potter 1971, Ten Have 2006, Lee 2017). Public health ethics emerged from concerns within contemporary bioethics about the health of individuals and populations, solidarity and justice, and natural and built environments; these concerns realign values of bioethics with environmental ethics by shifting from 'individual autonomy and the principle of least infringement to solidarity, interrelatedness, and the connection of human health to the health of the planet' (Lee 2017, p. 10). Reconnecting and nurturing these values can advance both fields and enhance health promotion and environmental protection.

Absent this reconnection, contemporary bioethics remains primarily concerned with individuals as recipients of medical and other types of healthcare (clinical ethics) and participants in health-related research (research ethics). Clinical ethics centers on relationships between provider and patient, and on individual and institutional responsibilities of providers to patients. Research ethics centers on protecting individual participants from unnecessary risks, wrongs, and harms of their participation in research studies and is increasingly attentive to protecting communities and populations. Public health ethics brings these together by focusing on activities aimed at improving community and population health through clinical and policy interventions and surveillance and research – activities that often improve the health of individuals within communities and populations.

Technological and pharmaceutical innovations that promote individual or population health are concerns of bioethics in its broadest sense. Research, development, and deployment of such innovations generate carbon emissions and waste and use resources in ways that harm environments even when less harmful approaches are feasible. This situation creates a conflict between the aim of health promotion by causing environmental damage. The aim of health promotion is accompanied, if not countered by, commercial interests that aim to increase profit and economic growth by developing, producing, and selling products required by health promotion such as those routinely used for screening, prevention, vaccination, or treatment. Production and sale of flu vaccines, equipment for mammography, and other widely used innovations promote health and generate profit for commercial interests.

Commercial interests in health promotion range from potential to blatant and embody conflicts of interest and conflicts of commitment that are not widely acknowledged or disclosed by healthcare institutions, practitioners, researchers, or ethicists although they permeate health promotion; that influential healthcare institutions are divesting from fossil fuels is indicative of growing awareness of, and concern about, such conflicts (Law *et al.* 2018). Through energy use and waste production, health promotion contributes to the severe and prevalent health impacts of climate change, and as they recognize this, healthcare institutions and providers are increasingly alarmed (Patz *et al.* 2014, Watts *et al.* 2018, Law *et al.* 2018, Swinburn *et al.* 2019).

Bioethical concern about using industrial levels of fossil fuels to promote health is growing because of the environmental impacts and health consequences of doing so. Bruce Jennings conceptualizes solidarity as a relational practice that can advance the engagement of health promotion with natural, built, and social environments including those implicated in climate change (Jennings 2015, Jennings and Dawson 2015, Jennings 2016, Solomon and Jennings 2017, Jennings 2018). This conception of solidarity embodies a motivation to stand up for, with, or as another and influences individual and collective wellbeing, actions, health, and healthcare (Solomon and Jennings 2017, Jennings 2018). Bioethics authors increasingly demonstrate willingness to reconnect with and embrace narratives of solidarity and relationships between human health and environments including those involving climate change (Schrader-Frechette 2002, Francis *et al.* 2005, Ten Have 2006, Ehrlich 2009, Dawson 2010, Resnik 2012, Macpherson 2013, Macpherson 2014, Bowen and Ebi 2015, Richie 2015, Valles 2015, Semplici 2016, Lee 2017). Environments provide resources that influence cultural identity and traditions as well as being essential to health, health promotion, and healthcare in different geographic contexts (Macpherson *et al.* 2016). Human encroachment on, and overuse of, environments and the resources they provide diminishes their sustainability and threatens human health and healthcare. Environmental protection is thus central to health promotion.

Responsibilities

Innovations and advancements in medicine have greatly improved human health over centuries. These include the development of antibiotics, vaccination, anesthesia, and sanitation systems that expand access to clean water, sewage systems, and waste collection and breakthroughs that have made cancers and non-communicable diseases more manageable, improved quality of life, and reduced mortality and morbidity (Weatherall *et al.* 2006). The exponential rates of such progress correspond with the growth of the healthcare industry and its expansive network of for-profit entities engaged in the business of providing health services (Ehrenreich and Ehrenreich 1970, Ehrenreich and Ehrenreich 1972). Commercial interests across the healthcare industry are associated with the overuse and fragmentation of services and overemphasis on expensive technology (Relman 1980). Values and policies that support market growth and elevate quarterly profits contribute to the medicalization of conditions that were not previously defined as diseases or disorders. Obesity, impotence, and pregnancy, for example, are now managed medically with costly services, technologies, and medications (Conrad and Leiter 2004).

Traditionally, the goals of medicine were to promote health by curing or managing disease and illness and helping patients return to their normal life (Daniels 1985). Commercial influences in healthcare have broadened this goal to encompass experimental interventions for human enhancement and personalized and precision medicine (Maturo 2012). Commercial influences have also increased the availability of direct-to-consumer (DTC) health products and services typically accessed without medical oversight or follow up such as genetic testing, mental health tools, neurostimulation devices, and heart rhythm monitors. DTC provides access to health promotion products and services that may not be otherwise accessible to them; it also encourages consumers to make purchases that are potentially unnecessary, expensive, or harmful, while increasing commercial profit. Health promotion and related spending in the USA grew to $3.65 trillion in 2018 (Sisko *et al.* 2019), an amount greater than many countries' GDP but yielding lower health outcomes than other high-income countries (Woolf and Aron 2013).

By increasing production and purchase of health promotion products, commercial interests compound conflicts between health promotion and environmental protection. Producing and selling these products may promote individual and population health but harms environments and diminishes rather than sustains environmental resources such as healthy food, air, water, and land. By consuming industrial levels of energy for heating, ventilation, air conditioning, anesthetics, and technologies, the healthcare industry including its' commercial interests release substantial quantities of greenhouse gas emissions and harm health in the short and long term (Thiel *et al.* 2015). Reliance on individually packaged pharmaceuticals and single use disposables such as syringes, sharps, and specula uses industrial levels of energy, water, and other resources involved in design, production, packaging, transportation, refrigeration, and disposal of such routine medical products, equipment, and services; in addition to emissions this releases radioactive, toxic, pharmaceutical, and electrical waste materials into land, water, and air (Zimmer and McKinley 2008).

Pharmaceutical waste includes analgesics, antibiotics, anticonvulsants, and contraceptives that contaminate ground water and drinking water, and damage aquatic life and ecosystems (Deo 2014). Imaging and drug delivery contribute to bioaccumulation of nanoparticles with unknown environmental and health impacts (Bystrzejewska-Piotrowska *et al.* 2009). Healthcare worsens air quality and may precipitate the onset and acute episodes of respiratory conditions through the release of emissions, particulate and smog pollution, acid rain, and stratospheric ozone depletion (British Lung Foundation 2018, Eckelman and Sherman 2016). Health promotion directly benefits patient and population health and simultaneously harms environments, patient, and population health. This conflict between the goals and outcomes of health promotion as conducted in wealthy countries today can be exacerbated, or minimized, by enacting environmental protections that instead promote health. Attention to extrinsic and intrinsic value of environments and environmental resources may guide decisionmakers to more accurately weigh and prioritize their use and protection and better serve the interests of health promotion.

The duty of rescue holds that healthcare providers, as institutions or individuals, should rescue one or more individuals from health harms or threats if that provider has the means to do so without significantly harming themselves (Osborne and Evans 1994, McKie and Richardson 2003). On a population rather than individual scale, this form of health promotion may also conflict with environmental protection. Criteria including proximity and relevant expertise should inform such determinations and when environmental harm seems disproportionately large may be countered by advocacy or other forms of environmental protection (Macpherson and Wynia 2017).

Synergy of health promotion and environmental protection

Having outlined conflicts between health promotion and environmental protection we now illustrate the synergy and compatibility of health promotion with environmental protection that derives from relationships between the respective goals and outcomes of these activities. Environments and their natural resources are intrinsic to the built environments in which we live, work, promote health, and access and deliver healthcare. They include Earth systems and the air, water, and geographies that these encompass. Unless human ingenuity can replace these on a global scale with something equivalent or better, which is at best unlikely, their protection is necessary for health and health promotion. Environments and their natural resources include protected forests and parks that serve as places of solace, inspiration, and recreation, to name a few. Protecting these places and access to them helps to preserve their capacity to reduce stress and enhance wellbeing, fitness, and creativity. The conflict between health promotion and environmental protection may be mitigated partly by reframing it in this way.

Climate change and the emissions that worsen it harm health, disrupts Earth systems, and seasonal patterns in ways that persist for decades or centuries. The health harms are sometimes direct for those with preexisting respiratory or other conditions and indirect for those injured, displaced, or afflicted by slower-onset psychiatric or psychological disorders (Watts *et al.* 2018). Health harms of such damage includes a serious threat to food security which are exacerbated by the agricultural industry through food-producing activities that significantly degrade and damage environments around the world – and reducing the capacity of environments to sustain food production (Swinburn *et al.* 2019). The agricultural industry promotes health by providing access to food, employment, and economic growth but simultaneously generates, globally, 30% of emissions, subsumes 40% of land and ecosystems that previously stored and mitigated greenhouse gases from the atmosphere as 'carbon sinks', and contributes to declining crop yields and quality in 30 countries (Swinburn *et al.* 2019).

As in healthcare, commercial interests in agriculture have conflicting aims: to provide healthy food and to increase its profits, wealth, and influence. The agricultural industry promotes individual and population health by providing food and simultaneously harms health by releasing much of our global emissions and using land and water resources wastefully and inequitably. Over decades and on a global scale, these activities have disrupted environments and seasonal patterns in ways that reduce agricultural productivity and facilitate emerging, re-emerging, and vector-borne diseases in areas previously inhospitable to their transmission (Watts *et al.* 2018, Patz *et al.* 2014). The agriculture and healthcare industries can and should accelerate constructive responses that reduce industrial, institutional, and national levels of emissions instead of continuing business as usual and contributing significantly to unacceptable health risks (Watts *et al.* 2018).

Medicine and nursing remain respected and trusted health professions with more influence than many others on patients, communities, and institutions. While promoting health and serving patients and populations, they and their employers generate large quantities of emissions through energy use, waste production, and procurement. Buildings in the UK's National Health Service (NHS) consume over US$500 million (£410 million) worth of energy and account for 24% of the carbon footprint of the entire NHS (NHS Sustainable Development Unit 2020).

The investigation and exposure by healthcare professionals of links between tobacco use and cancer, and resultant regulations on the tobacco industry, grew out of a professional mandate to promote health, which includes protection against significant health threats. Likewise, professionals and their institutions should 'help society move away from fossil fuels and accelerate the transition to renewable energy' (Law *et al.* 2018). Healthcare professionals and institutions are committed to and capable of promoting health. They can and should engage in and advocate for changes in their workplaces that promote energy efficiency improvements, increase fresh and locally produced foods in their food services, and integrate ecofriendly practices and products into housekeeping, transportation, and other institutional practices (Macpherson and Wynia 2017). Doing so directly promotes health while protecting environments and the environmental resources essential for health.

The healthcare industry can promote health while conserving energy and related costs in many ways including architectural initiatives designed to increase proximity of patients and staff to green spaces which is in hospital settings to facilitate physical activity, accelerate recovery, and reduce pain, aggression, mental fatigue, and staff burnout (Sadler et al. 2011). Large amounts of energy and landfill waste can be safely reduced by modifying procedures for hospital-based cannulation and intravenous antibiotic preparation (Bajgoric et al. 2014), disposal of unused pharmaceuticals (Maughan et al. 2014), recycling of medical equipment (Kwakye et al. 2010), and other approaches (Health Research and Educational Trust 2014).

Healthcare professionals and their institutions have many such opportunities to conserve energy and reduce emissions. Reasons to do so include both moral responsibilities as individuals and professional responsibilities stemming from unique knowledge, influence, resources, trusted positions, and socioeconomic status. Those who fail to act on these responsibilities are accepting and supporting the status quo production of emissions by their institutions. Healthcare professionals are better positioned than many to champion carbon reduction and control and are blameworthy for failing to counter background conditions in ways that reduce the harms of emissions (Shockley 2017).

Even when providing necessary goods and services, industries and institutions routinely use and damage environments and natural resources on the grounds that they are boosting employment and economic development while providing needed goods and services. Using public or environmental resources, infrastructure, or services without replenishing, maintaining, or compensating for this use is a form of free-riding that imposes moral responsibilities on those who do so, particularly on those who gain commercially or at the expense of others from doing so (Hughes 2014, Macpherson 2019a). These responsibilities are heightened when their own institutional policies and practices have large, widespread, and severe consequences such as those of environmental degradation and loss.

It is in the public interest to protect the health and resilience of environments and resources from overuse or destruction caused by economic and commercial interests (Norton 2017). Industrial use of natural environments and resources has pronounced social and ecological costs that are avoidable or can be made less harmful by integrating them into economic policy and development, calculating them appropriately, providing compensation, and protecting against further loss of environments and carbon sinks (Jamieson 2014, Schor 2010). Industries and institutions have capacity to reduce their own emissions and curtail and repair damages. Existing governmental and intergovernmental regulation and governance of their activities do not adequately monitor or require changes but industrial and institutional leaders have responsibilities and choices about whether and how to reduce and repair damages they contribute to, or compensate for, free-riding on public goods and environments.

Our industrial practices, priorities, and values emerged in a low tech and sparsely populated world that has changed significantly over recent decades and should be recalibrated to preserve the capacity of Earth systems, environments, and resources for present and future people globally (Garvey 2008). The primary cause of climate change is industrial release of emissions during the production and distribution of energy, safe water, and food. That industries profit economically from this release – and have greater capacity than those with less wealth, resources, and influence to reduce emissions – warrants greater attention among institutional, corporate, and governmental leaders. These leaders have moral responsibilities to adequately compensate for their use of natural resources, damages to environments, and failure to significantly reduce their own emissions (Macpherson 2019b).

Given the goals of healthcare, claims of and calls for health promotion are hypocritical unless they involve strategies and policies that explicitly protect environments and natural resources. Health promotion harms the environment but can be conducted less harmfully if those conducting it contribute, with others, to protecting, maintaining, and replenishing the resources used. Cristina Richie's construct of Green Bioethics describes why and how healthcare can improve health while conserving environments and natural resources through, among others, nurturing innovations that manage or prevent medical disorders rather than advancing optional or 'luxury' interventions linked with enhancement or fertility (Richie 2019). The healthcare industry can safely, effectively, and presumably with limited economic loss, integrate energy and waste conservation into its routine practices.

Industries and their institutions should move to adopt more environmentally friendly policies and practices immediately. How best to do this is an empirical question with normative components regarding which tradeoffs result in the best options. The healthcare industry is by nature concerned with health promotion and should acknowledge its responsibility to modify policies and practices in ways that reduce ongoing environmental damage. Doing so is challenging but feasible and morally required given global population and its projected growth.

Three radical examples

Industrial and institutional support is essential to such initiatives and promoting human and environmental health now and in the future. We now offer radical examples of health promotion projects supported by many in healthcare and health research to demonstrate the potential for the healthcare industry and its institutions to partner on both promoting health while protecting environments, despite the complexity and challenges to doing so.

1. Saving people and the environment by creating fewer people

The tension between human health promotion and environmental protection is due, in large part, to the number of humans on the planet. Total environmental impact is a product of individual environmental impact times the number of individuals. A rather distressing way to put the tension is to note that rescuing people – not to mention promoting their full, healthy lives, defined by plentiful, nutritious food consumption and energy-emitting activities – strains the environment simply by increasing the burden of use. If people die or are so poor or unhealthy as to limit their environmental impact, this benefits an overstressed planet.

The tension between human and environmental health, then, is a consequence of *overpopulation*. This is not yet a problem of raw numbers of people on the planet, but of some number of people using resources at some particular level. Climate change is caused by some number of people emitting at various levels. If we are unable to successfully decrease their emissions fast enough to prevent massive harm to the environment, and then to humans, there is another variable to which we could apply pressure: the number of emitters. That is to say: both human and environmental health could be promoted by reducing the number of people on the planet.

One way to respond to this suggestion would be to admit that promoting human health harms the environment and so we should stop promoting human health – at least in certain circumstances. Perhaps we should stop trying to cure people of diseases since they will be too environmentally expensive or, worse yet, perhaps we should stop trying to promote the health of the world's poorest and worst off since they currently use precious few resources and increasing their health would lead them to be environmentally expensive like us globally wealthy citizens.

Although these sorts of suggestions do in fact respond to the tension, they are also clearly problematic: the latter because it is strikingly unfair to ask the world's worst-off to carry the burden of saving the earth's environment and the former because being sick does not necessarily make death any less frightening or bad. But what these unhelpful suggestions *do* get right is the following two points: (i) once someone exists, consuming resources is important for their health, which is why the world's poorest need to consume more; and (ii) the death rate is one way to control the size of the human population. Recognizing these two points then makes clear why it is much preferable to resolve the tension between human and environmental health promotion by reducing the number of people who come into existence rather than by giving some of them very few resources or allowing some to die.

Human and environmental health, in other words, are both promoted by reducing the total fertility rate until human population and consumption are at a level such that they do not create the tension under investigation. Although this idea is disconcerting to many, and has been taboo for much of recent history, it is beginning to enter the ethics literature explicitly as a result of today's looming environmental catastrophes. For just a brief selection, Colin Hickey, Travis Rieder, and Jake Earl discuss the need for fertility reduction policies (Hickey *et al*. 2016) and immigration management (Earl *et al*. 2017) in order to meet morally required climate mitigation efforts. Conly (2015) promotes the global adoption of a one-child policy for the same reason. Rieder (2016) and Hedberg (2020) both argue that such considerations should actually lead individuals to change their procreative behaviors as a result. The views under consideration, in short, are that people should have small families and policies should encourage them to do so. The frame of population-level bioethics makes explicit that these are public health arguments for interventions that both protect the natural environment, and that by doing so protect human health.

Although the discussion of fertility reduction practices and policies tend to make people uncomfortable, calling to mind racist and eugenicist motives or the human-rights abuses suffered during China's Family Planning Policy, all of the aforementioned authors argue that fertility reduction can be achieved permissibly. Although coercion and bias are, of course, possible in this domain (as in many others), they are not necessary. Indeed, many justice- and autonomy-enhancing interventions are actually fertility-reducing interventions. This is especially true when considering the impact of providing healthcare, access to family planning, and the education and empowerment of women and young girls anywhere that it is lacking. These efforts alone have a dramatic fertility-reducing effect. Significant advances can also be made through social marketing campaigns and, where possible, utilizing positive and negative incentives such as removing child tax credits for the wealthy (Hickey *et al.* 2016). None of these interventions are particularly coercive and certainly none of them involve human rights abuses or are inherently biased although care would need to be taken in implementation.

The size of the human population is controlled through the relationship between the birth rate and the death rate, and the impact of the human population on the environment is mediated by the consumption and emission level of individuals. Since increasing the death rate and taking away health-promoting opportunities to consume and emit are not ethically promising interventions, modifying the birth rate may well be the best opportunity for relieving the tension between human and environmental health promotion. Reducing the birth rate is one way to promote health and protect environments.

2. Promoting human and environmental health by transforming the food system

Humans cannot be healthy without nutritious and uncontaminated food. Our health, emotions, and sense of wellbeing are affected by the type and quality of food we eat and the social context in which it is prepared and consumed. The complex web of activities involving food production, processing, transport, and consumption is called the 'food system' and includes related governance, economics, sustainability, waste, and impacts on environments as well as on individual and population health (Oxford Martin Program 2020). Vast environmental spaces and resources are used by the food system to produce and deliver food around the world. The healthcare industry is involved in evaluating and making nutritional recommendations and in delivering food to patients and employees. Agriculture, transportation, and energy industries are central to the food system given their contributions to producing, storing, processing, packaging, marketing, and selling food and disposing of food waste. Human health is affected by these and other industries.

Foods vary in calories, nutrition, and the environmental resources used in their production. There is global concern about growing demand and declining food quantity and quality. Globally, the food system overproduces foods with limited nutrition, fails to equitably make nutritious food accessible and affordable for all, generates roughly 30% of global emissions and climate change, and is unnecessarily burdensome to Earth's capacity to feed the projected 10 billion people who will be alive in 2050 (Swinburn *et al.* 2019). Ideally, the endpoints of the food system are global consumption of adequate dietary quantity and quality of food and food production that does no further damage to Earth's geophysical systems or environments (Swinburn *et al.* 2019). Feeding 10 billion people accordingly requires transformation of the global food system in line with scientific and clinical evidence and supported by soft and hard policies (Swinburn *et al.* 2019). Failure to transform it will have global and regional impacts such as raising food prices and food scarcity. Food scarcity and insecurity are known to precipitate social conditions of displacement, unrest, and sometimes violent conflict and political upheaval – conditions that undermine individual and population health, raising demand for healthcare, and overburden healthcare institutions.

Rising emissions and manifestations of climate change harm environments and environmental resources that are essential to health, health promotion, and healthcare. Our growing global population requires growing quantities of healthy food and makes environmental protection an ethical imperative. Healthcare industries, institutions, and professionals have professional responsibilities to care for patients and populations. They violate these responsibilities by ignoring social or environmental conditions that harm health locally or globally.

The agricultural industry similarly has a responsibility to produce and make accessible uncontaminated, nutritious, and affordable food globally. It can and should change its policies and procedures in ways that make healthy food accessible to everyone including the least well- off. Doing so would contribute to economic and political stability of populations and nations and maintain environmental and social conditions in which the agricultural industry itself can continue to prosper. It would also support social justice, promote health, protect environments, and sustain the capacity to profit commercially. From a civic perspective, all industries and governments arguably share such responsibilities and should support this transformation of the food system despite the economic and political challenges that doing so poses. These are outweighed by global health benefits and their local and global economic consequences. Transforming the food system to promote health and protect environments requires reducing agricultural food waste and energy use; limiting additional agricultural land, water, and fertilizer use; reducing dietary consumption of sugar and red meat; and increasing consumption of fruits, vegetables, and legumes (Swinburn *et al.* 2019). Transforming the food system accordingly is a promising way to promote health and protect environments.

3. Promoting human health by genetically modifying mosquitoes

Mosquito control is essential to promote health but often conflicts with protecting the environment. Mosquitoes transmit numerous diseases to human beings including malaria, dengue fever, and West Nile fever. Over 200 million people worldwide contract malaria each year and about 400,000 die from the disease (World Health Organization 2019). Controlling mosquito populations is the most effective way of preventing mosquito-borne diseases. However, some methods of mosquito control can cause significant environmental damage (World Health Organization 2014). For example, draining mosquito breeding grounds such as wetlands can destroy habitats, disrupt ecosystems, and reduce biodiversity. Spraying pesticides can have harmful effects on non-target species such as insects, birds, fish, and other aquatic organisms. Additionally, mosquitoes may become resistant to pesticides (Resnik 2012).

DDT (dichlorodiphenyltrichloroethane) is an insecticide highly effective at killing mosquitoes. DDT was used widely in the 1940s and 1950s to control mosquito populations until research 1960s demonstrated that it is toxic to birds, cats, and fish. Over 150 countries have banned DDT, but several African nations still use it to control malaria because of its effectiveness. Although scientists initially thought that moderate use of DDT did not pose any significant risks to human beings, studies in the last few decades have shown that DDT exposure can increase the risk of premature birth, low birth weight, and some types of cancer (Carson 1962, Resnik 2012). Other types of pesticides used to control mosquitoes such a malathion, naled, phenothrin, permethrin, and pyrethrins can also have adverse effects on the environment (Resnik 2012). As an alternative way of preventing mosquito-borne diseases, scientists have developed two different methods for using genetically modified (GM) mosquitoes, but both methods pose risks to the environment.

The first method, which has been tested in the field, suppresses populations of mosquitoes that transmit a specific disease, such as dengue fever, by introducing a lethal mutation that kills offspring before they reach adulthood (Carvalho et al. 2015). The primary environmental risk of this method is that it could it disrupt the food web by drastically reducing mosquito populations (Meghani and Kuzma 2018). If species that prey on mosquitoes in these ecosystems find alternative sources of food then environmental disruption may be minimal.

The second method introduces a gene into the mosquito population that prevents them from carrying or transmitting a targeted disease such as malaria. It has only been tested in the laboratory and uses a gene drive system to increase the prevalence of the gene in the population (Hammond and Galizi 2017). A gene drive is a relatively new technology designed to alter the genetics of a target species. It may have long term consequences for the target species because genetic material is transmitted to future generations. It may also affect species that prey on mosquitoes in unknown and unanticipated ways and potentially disrupt the food web. It raises ethical questions involving risks, limitations, and responsibilities. First, for example, genetically modifying mosquitoes with a gene drive might not work as intended and could cause genetic changes that make the mosquitoes more likely to transmit diseases to humans. Second, the targeted pathogen might evolve in response to changes in the mosquito population and become more virulent or deadly. Third, horizontal gene transfer could move the gene drive system from the mosquito population into other populations and have unpredictable genetic and phenotypic effects on a range of species. Although horizontal gene transfer is rare, the consequences for human or environmental health are unknown and potentially significant.

Mosquito control poses difficult ethical challenges for public health agencies, researchers, and the public because the conflict between promoting human health and protecting the environment is unavoidable. Moreover, there are potential off target impacts of chemical and other interventions that may directly or indirectly affect humans. For example, the World Health Organization decision in 2006 to endorse limited use of DDT in nations facing severe malaria problems divided public health researchers and professionals. While many agree with the WHO that using DDT was necessary to prevent malaria in some unique circumstances, others hold the opposite view.

GM mosquitoes may pose less of a risk to the environment than other methods of preventing mosquito-borne diseases but pose potential risks that are not well understood. Further research is needed to better understand to the benefits, risks, and limitations of using GM mosquitoes to control mosquito-borne diseases. Research and interventions that release GM mosquitoes into the environment raise important issues pertaining to social justice and democracy because people who live near the release sites will likely be more impacted by those mosquitoes than those living further away. While there is widespread agreement that researchers and public health officials should consult local communities prior to releasing GM mosquitoes, important issues still need to be resolved such as how to engage the public and communities fairly and effectively (Resnik 2019).

Health promotion involves efforts to reduce and control transmission of mosquito-borne and other vector-borne diseases to humans. Disease vectors are part of the environment. Destroying, displacing, or genetically modifying mosquitoes and other vectors may disrupt the environment, ecosystems, and the food web. For regions with severe morbidity and mortality due to mosquito-borne disease such as malaria or Zika, the risks and harms of GM mosquitoes must be balanced against the short and long term consequences for human health and the environment in those and other regions. Technological innovations to control mosquitoes and other disease vectors, and other serious threats to human health may be valuable and may be harmful. Research is therefore needed to help identify and understand the potential off target impacts of any new technological innovation. GM mosquitoes are an example of health promotion that conflicts with environmental protection. Ethically, it is unclear when or whether the environmental risk of GM mosquitoes, and consequences for human health, are outweighed by the benefits.

Conclusion

Health promotion does not have to conflict with environmental protection. Industries, their leaders, and institutions have opportunities and means to protect against environmental disruption and harm, and have responsibilities to do so because it contributes to sustaining health, environments, food security, social stability, and their own commercial and economic gains. The agricultural industry with its global influence and intense use of environmental resources has a unique responsibility to sustain and provide access to healthy food by transforming the food system. The healthcare industry with its commitment to health and health promotion has a particular responsibility to reduce its own energy use and waste production without compromising healthcare standards.

Slowing the global birthrate, transforming the food system, and GM mosquitoes each aim to promote health. The global birthrate can be reduced without infringing on reproductive choice or violating human rights if social, political, and other mechanisms deliver relevant information and contraceptive products. Reducing the global birthrate protects the environment by reducing demand for and use of its resources. The many components of the food system can be transformed to better protect environments by using less water and energy and generating less waste if its industrial leaders are willing to sacrifice short term quarterly gains and adopt environmentally sustainable policies and practices. This requires motivation, courage, and creativity, and demonstrates that health promotion and environmental protection can be reciprocal and symbiotic rather than in conflict. Technological approaches to health promotion including GM mosquitos may conflict with environmental protection because of their unanticipated and harmful off target impacts on environments, including energy use and the generation of unnecessary emissions and waste.

Health, health promotion, and healthcare cannot exist when environments and environmental resources are misused or undervalued. Their value must be integrated into policies, practices, regulations, and governance by the governments, industries, and institutions charged with sustaining health, economic stability, and wellbeing. Health promotion does not have to conflict with environmental protection, although it may in some situations. The conflicts of concern for health promotion are the ongoing and extensive environmental damage and destruction by industries, particularly those that do so while promoting health or their own commercial gain, and the abrogation of related responsibility. It is time for industries, institutions, and governments to re-think their values, priorities, policies, and practices.

Acknowledgment

We thank David B. Resnik for significant contributions to this paper.

Disclosure statement

No potential conflict of interest was reported by the author(s).

ORCID

Cheryl C. Macpherson http://orcid.org/0000-0002-2368-2089
Travis N. Rieder http://orcid.org/0000-0002-2919-8634

References

Bajgoric, S., et al., 2014. Sustainability in clinical skills teaching. *The clinical teacher*, 11 (4), 243–246.
Bowen, K.J., and Ebi, K.L., 2015. Governing the health risks of climate change: towards multi-sector responses. *Current opinion in environmental sustainability*, 12, 80–85.
British Lung Foundation, 2018. Toxic air at the door of the NHS [online]. Available from: https://www.blf.org.uk/take-action/campaign/nhs-toxic-air-report [Last Accessed 20 May, 2020].
Bystrzejewska-Piotrowska, G., Golimowski, J., and Urban, P.L., 2009. Nanoparticles: their potential toxicity, waste and environmental management. *Waste management*, 29 (9), 2587–2595.
Carson, R., 1962. *Silent Spring*. St Charles, IL: Houghton Mifflin Company.
Carvalho, D.O., et al., 2015. Suppression of a field population of Aedes aegypti in Brazil by sustained release of transgenic male mosquitoes. *PLos neglected tropical diseases*, 9 (7), e0003864.
Center for Disease Control. 2019. One Health [online]. Available from: https://www.cdc.gov/onehealth/index.html [Accessed 11 Mar 2019].
Conly, S., 2015. *One child: do we have a right to more?* Oxford: Oxford University Press.
Conrad, P., and Leiter, V., 2004. Medicalization, markets and consumers. *Journal of health and social behavior*, 45, 158–176.
Daniels, N., 1985. *Just health care*. New York: Cambridge University Press.
Dawson, A., 2010. The future of bioethics: three Dogmas and a Cup of Hemlock. *Bioethics*, 24 (5), 218–225.
Deo, R.P., 2014. Pharmaceuticals in the Surface water of the USA: a review. *Current environmental health Reports*, 1 (2), 113–122.
Dupras, C., Ravitsky, V., and Williams-Jones, B., 2014. Epigenetics and the environment in bioethics. *Bioethics*, 28 (7), 327–334.

Earl, J., Hickey, C., and Rieder, T.N., 2017. Fertility, immigration, and the fight against climate change. *Bioethics*, 31 (8), 582–589.

Eckelman, M.J., and Sherman, J., 2016. Environmental impacts of the U.S. health care system and effects on public health. *PLOS ONE*, 11 (6), e0157014.

Ehrenreich, B., and Ehrenreich, J., 1970. The medical industrial complex. *NY Review of Books*, 14.

——., 1972. The American health empire: power, profits and politics. *Science and society*, 36 (1), 95–99.

Ehrlich, P.R., 2009. Ecoethics: now central to all ethics. *Journal of bioethical inquiry*, 6 (4), 417–436.

Francis, L.P., et al., 2005. How infectious diseases got left out–and what this omission might have meant for bioethics. *Bioethics*, 19 (4), 307–322.

Garvey, J., 2008. *The ethics of climate change: right and Wrong in a Warming world*. New York City, NY: Continuum Press.

Hammond, A.M., and Galizi, R., 2017. Gene drives to fight malaria: current state and future directions. *Pathogens and global health*, 111 (8), 412–423.

Health Research and Educational Trust. 2014. Environmental sustainability in hospitals: the value of efficiency. Available from: http://www.hpoe.org/Reports-HPOE/ashe-sustainability-report-FINAL.pdf [Last Accessed 20 March 2020].

Hedberg, T., 2020. *The environmental impact of overpopulation: The ethics of procreation*. London: Routledge.

Hickey, C., Rieder, T.N., and Earl, J., 2016. Population Engineering and the Fight against climate change. *Social theory and practice*, 42 (4), 845–870.

Hughes, R.C., 2014. Justifying community benefit requirements in international research. *Bioethics*, 28(8): 397-404.

Jamieson, D., 2014. *Reason in a dark time: why the struggle against climate change Failed—and what it means for our future*. Oxford: Oxford University Press.

Jennings, B., 2015. Relational liberty revisited: membership, solidarity and a public health ethics of place. *Public health ethics*, 8 (1), 7–17.

——., 2016. Reconceptualizing autonomy: a relational turn in bioethics. *Hastings Center Report*, 46 (3), 11–16.

——., 2018. Solidarity and care as relational practices. *Bioethics*, 32 (9), 553–561.

Jennings, B., and Dawson, A., 2015. Solidarity in the moral imagination of bioethics. *Hastings Center Report*, 45 (5), 31–38.

Kwakye, G., et al., 2010. Commentary: a call to go green in health care by reprocessing medical equipment. *Academic medicine*, 85 (3), 398–400.

Lang, T., and Rayner, G., 2012. Ecological public health: the twenty-first century's big idea? An essay by Tim Lang and Geof Rayner. *BMJ*, 345, e5466.

Law, A., et al., 2018. Medical organisations must divest from fossil fuels. *BMJ*, 363, k5163.

Lee, L.M., 2017. A Bridge Back to the future: public health ethics, bioethics, and environmental ethics. *The American Journal of bioethics*, 17 (9), 5–12.

Macpherson, C.C., 2013. Climate change is a bioethics problem. *Bioethics*, 27 (6), 305–308. doi:10.1111/bioe.12029.

——., 2014. Climate change matters. *Journal of medical ethics*, 40 (4), 288–290.

——., 2019a. Research ethics guidelines and moral obligations to developing countries: capacity-building and benefits. *Bioethics,* 33: 399–405.

——., 2019b. Energy, emissions, and public health ethics. In: A Mastroianni, N Kass, and J Kahn, eds. *Oxford Handbook of public health ethics*. New York, NY: Oxford University Press, 739–754.

Macpherson, C.C., Bidaisee, S., and Macpherson, C.N.L., 2016. Environmental harms in distant polar regions and small island developing states. In: C.C. Macpherson eds, *Bioethical Insights into values and policy: climate change and health*. New York, NY: Springer Press, 127–142.

Macpherson C.C. and Wynia M., 2017. Speaking up: are health professionals obligated to advocate for actions to reduce the health risks of climate change. *AMA Journal of ethics* 19, 1202–1210. Available from: http://journalofethics.ama-assn.org/2017/12/pdf/msoc1-1712.pdf

Maturo, A., 2012. Medicalization: current concept and future directions in a bionic society. *Mens sana monographs*, 10 (1), 122–133.

Maughan, D., et al., 2014. What psychiatrists should know about environmental sustainability and what they should be doing about it. *International psychiatry*, 11 (2), 27–30.

McKie, J., and Richardson, J., 2003. The rule of rescue. *Social science & medicine*, 56 (12), 2407–2419.

Meghani, Z., and Kuzma, J., 2018. Regulating animals with gene drive systems: lessons from the regulatory assessment of a genetically engineered mosquito. *Journal of responsible innovation*, 5 (sup1), S203–S222.

NHS England and Public Health England. 2020. Sustainable development unit. Energy and carbon management [online]. Available from: https://www.sduhealth.org.uk/ [Last Accessed 18 Mar, 2020].

Norton, B.G., 2017. Sustainability as the multigenerational public interest. In: S.M. Gardiner, and A. Thompson, eds. *Oxford Handbook of environmental ethics*. New York, NY: Oxford University Press, 355–366.

Osborne, M., and Evans, T.W., 1994. Allocation of resources in intensive care: a transatlantic perspective. *The lancet*, 343 (8900), 778–780.

Oxford Martin Program on the Future of Food. Available from: https://www.futureoffood.ox.ac.uk/what-food-system [Last Accessed 14 March 2020].

Patz JA, et al., 2014. Climate change: challenges and opportunities for global health. *JAMA*, 312(15):1565–1580. doi:10.1001/jama.2014.13186

Potter, V.R., 1971. *Bioethics: Bridge to the future*. Upper Sadle River, NJ: Prentice-Hall.

Relman, A.S., 1980. The New medical-industrial complex. *New England Journal of medicine*, 303 (17), 963–970.

Resnik, D.B., 2009. Human health and the environment: In Harmony or in conflict? *Health care analysis: HCA : journal of health philosophy and policy*, 17 (3), 261–276.

——., 2012. *Environmental health ethics*. Cambridge: Cambridge University Press.

——., 2019. Two unresolved issues in community engagement for field trials of genetically modified mosquitoes. *Pathogens and global health*, 113 (5), 238–245.

Richie, C., 2015. Laudato Si', Catholic health care, and climate change. *Health care ethics*, 23, 3.

——., 2019. *Principles of green bioethics: sustainability in health care*. East Lansing, MI: Michigan State University Press.

Rieder, T., 2016. *Toward a small family ethic: how overpopulation and climate change are affecting the Morality of Procreation*. New York City, NY: Springer.

Sadler, B.L., et al., 2011. Fable hospital 2.0: the business case for building better health care facilities. *The Hastings Center report*, 41 (1), 13–23.

Schor, J.B., 2010. *Plenitude: The New economics of true wealth*. New York City, NY: Penguin Press.

Semplici, S., 2016. Global bioethics as social bioethics. *In*: A. Bagheri, J.D. Moreno and S. Semplici, eds. *Global bioethics: the impact of the Unesco International bioethics Committee*New York City, NY: Springer Nature, 57–71.

Shockley, K., 2017. Responsibility. In: S.M. Gardiner, and A. Thompson, ed. *Oxford Handbook of environmental ethics*. New York, NY: Oxford University Press, 265–275.

Shrader-Frechette, K.S., 2002. *Environmental justice: creating equality, reclaiming democracy*. New York: Oxford University Press.

Sisko, A.M., et al., 2019. National health Expenditure projections, 2018–27: economic and demographic trends drive spending and enrollment growth. *Health affairs*, 38 (3), 491–501.

Solomon, M.Z., and Jennings, B., 2017. Bioethics and populism: how should our field respond? *Hastings center report*, 47 (2), 11–16.

Swinburn, B.A., et al., 2019. The global syndemic of obesity, undernutrition, and climate change: the Lancet Commission report. *The lancet*, 393 (10173), 791–846.

Ten Have, H., 2006. The activities of UNESCO in the Area of ethics. *Kennedy Institute of ethics journal*, 16 (4), 333–351.

Thiel, C.L., et al., 2015. Environmental impacts of surgical procedures: life cycle assessment of hysterectomy in the United States. *Environmental science & technology*, 49 (3), 1779–1786.

Valles, S.A., 2015. Bioethics and the Framing of climate change's health risks. *Bioethics*, 29 (5), 334–341.

Watts, N., et al., 2018. The 2018 report of the Lancet Countdown on health and climate change: shaping the health of nations for centuries to come. *The lancet*, 392 (10163), 2479–2514.

Weatherall, D., et al., 2006. Science and technology for disease control: past, present, and future. *In*: D.T. Jamison, J.G. Breman, A.R. Measham, eds. *Disease control priorities in developing countries*. Washington, DC: World Bank. https://www.ncbi.nlm.nih.gov/books/NBK11740/. [Last Accessed 20 May, 2020].

Woolf, S.H., and Aron, L.Y., 2013. The US health disadvantage relative to other high-income countries: findings from a national research Council/institute of medicine report. *JAMA*, 309 (8), 771–772.

World Health Organization. 2014. Guidance Framework for Testing of Genetically Modified Mosquitoes. Available at: https://www.who.int/tdr/publications/year/2014/guide-fmrk-gm-mosquit/en/ [Last Accessed 18 Mar, 2020].

——.. 2016. What is health promotion? Available from: http://www.who.int/features/qa/health-promotion/en/ [Last Accessed 31 Jan, 2019].

——.. 2019. Malaria. Available from: https://www.who.int/malaria/en/ [Last Accessed: October 9, 2019].

Zimmer, C., and McKinley, D., 2008. New approaches to pollution prevention in the healthcare industry. *Journal of cleaner production*, 16 (6), 734–742.

Bioethics and Environmental Ethics: The Story of the Human Body as a Natural Ecosystem

Zoe-Athena Papalois

Kyriaki-Barbara Papalois

Is there a parallel between climate change and our body's temperature or non-compliance and failure to act on global warming? This paper proposes a model which describes the human body as part of Nature's ecosystem. By utilising the power of observation to identify a problem, environmental and applied ethics can guide action and instigate change, not only to change the predicted plot of climate change, but also the wellbeing of humans in life's story. Through a discussion on human autonomy and lessons learned from the past, earth's inhabitants can identify a balance between beneficence and non-maleficence for themselves and our planet.

Introduction: empirical medicine

The catalytic importance of empirical observation has been demonstrated throughout the history of Medicine. In Ancient Greece, Hippocrates, the father of modern medicine pioneered the concept of empirical observation. Discerning parallels between nature and the human body, Hippocrates developed a diagnostic theory and therapeutic principles. By demonstrating that disease has a natural history, Hippocrates' work was pivotal in shifting the predominantly superstitious mentalities that dominated contemporary thinking, from supernatural to natural causes.

In the 1700s, Edward Jenner noted that milkmaids who contracted cowpox had a reduced incidence of contracting deadly smallpox (Stewart and Devlin 2006). After the introduction of inoculation, vaccination flourished, with smallpox being declared an eradicated disease by the World Health Organization (WHO) in 1980 (Weiss and Esparza 2015). After Jenner's discovery, many other vaccines against devastating diseases followed, which routinely save millions of lives today.

In the Victorian era, Ignaz Semmelweis observed that women during childbirth often died of puerperal fever when medical students and young doctors assisted with the labour. However, this did not occur when the nurses were present at the birth (Ataman et al. 2013). He hypothesised this disparity in death rate was due medical students visiting the cadaver lab prior to hospital ward rounds, which led to a transmission of disease. In turn he postulated that carbolic acid would reduce the incidence of puerperal fever.

In the modern era, empirical medicine is the standard. The WHO has been tirelessly fighting to bridge the gaps in health inequality around the world and pioneer initiatives to aid in the eradication of disease, as well as the prevention of illness, and better quality of life worldwide. Annually, there are Awareness Days for specific conditions, increasing health literacy about medical topics and informing behaviour to improve general health. Systematic reviews and meta-analyses of research collate and summarise evidence to inform healthcare professionals and practitioners of new developments annually, thereby informing evidence-based medicine (Purden et al. 2013). This information informs patient care practices.

Every medical consultation or interaction commences with a medical history. Clinicians attempt to understand how a patient's anatomy and physiology has evolved and which variables have contributed to this evolution. Natural history is more than uncovering aetiology. It is about deciding where the patient is going by knowing where they have already been. Every patient's destination will be different. For example, while a surgeon may know the anatomical components that constitute a hand, the way that the patient before them has used their hand during their lifetime and what they hope to use it for in the future dramatically alter the procedural approach and the stakes. Simultaneously, the patient's goals can direct the preservation of health.

The preservation of health depends on a delicate balance of physiological processes, known as 'homeostasis'. This remarkable concept describes the human body's intrinsic tendency towards equilibrium. A change in one direction elicits a response in the opposite direction, restoring harmony. An excessive shift results in a change that cannot be compensated. This imbalance results in illness. In many ways, there are parallels between approaches to understanding climate change and approaches to health.

Observational climate

The powerful use of observation has elucidated parallels between our health and behaviour with the environment. Observation allows for introspection, which is the first step to responsibility. In the discipline of environmental science, progress was stagnant for centuries because the causative relationship between human activity and climate change was met with scepticism. As a result, climate change was considered an inevitable state and 'red-flags,' such as the increase in atmospheric temperature, melting of polar ice-caps, and rise in sea level were analogous to 'medically unexplained symptoms'. Efforts to dismiss the problem downplayed the severity of climate change by framing it in the context of cyclical changes in the Earth's temperature that have occurred since the beginning of time (Steffen *et al.* 2015). Such ignorance is dangerous because it diminishes human responsibility and implies a lack of effort to fully comprehend the issue.

Humans cannot change the weather. They can only adapt to it. In the medical analogy, this is akin to a 'symptomatic management' treatment approach. While therapeutic, this approach is not curative. An extension of this paradigm is the knowledge that weather is a symptom of climate and climate is significantly influenced by human actions. In effect, humans need to find the root cause of climate change. In the search, humanity might find that they are partially responsible for the problem, which we can amend through action. However, there may be additional factors beyond our control.

A demonstrative analogy is found in mental health. 'Weather' corresponds to the normal, and sometimes temperamental, fluctuations in mood that everyone experiences. By analogy, 'climate' refers to the baseline emotional state. This is what clinically distinguishes 'depressive disorder,' requiring treatment, from 'sadness,' which is temporary and self-limiting (Malla *et al.* 2015). The same parallelism can be applied to virtually any disease. Manifesting symptoms are a warning sign of an underlying disturbance in the body's 'climate'. For example, a fever demonstrates a rise in baseline body temperature. This is indicative of an inflammatory response, triggered by an invasion of a pathogenic microorganism, which the body has been unable to expel or defeat.

In another example, destroying the planet is akin to an act of self-harm, which is a symptom of an internal self-conflict stemming from a wounded heart, crying out for help. Similar mentalities are seen in self-provoked diseases, such as pulmonary disease as a result of smoking, liver failure induced by chronic alcohol excess, or psychosis induced by recreational drug use. The common denominator in each of these examples is the prevalence of immediate gratification over consideration for long term consequences. The exploitation of natural resources meets demands of consumers, but comes at a long term cost.

Like climate, human health is not an independent entity, existing in isolation. Rather, a healthy state is a product of processes and choices. Some of the determinants of health are within human control, whilst other are not. Matters are further complicated by the fact that a 'healthy state' is not a discrete quality, categorised as either present or absent. 'Health' encompasses a spectrum of oscillating states. The Intergovernmental Panel on Climate Change concluded that climate change is a multifactorial issue, however, the greatest contributor is human activity and fossil fuel consumption (Intergovernmental Panel on Climate Change 2001). Climate is not independent from actions. Nor can we say that humans are discrete entities exempt from the laws of nature.

Nature: a mirror of the human body

Four examples highlight how the processes of nature mirror those of the human body: Type II diabetes, wound regeneration, entropy, and biodiversity. In these examples, the first two start in the body and are applicable to nature. In the latter two examples, the converse approach is taken. In aggregate, the examples are illustrative of the connections between climate and health.

Type 2 diabetes is an evolved inability to regulate blood sugar levels. The normal homeostatic mechanism, by which insulin release counters the rise in blood glucose, becomes fatigued. In the place of homeostasis, the body adapts to a 'new normal'. This is analogous to the greenhouse effect – the main contributor towards the climate change phenomenon. The exponential rise in greenhouse gas emissions over time has led to a progressive increase in atmospheric temperature because their cumulative impact far exceeds the atmosphere's compensatory mechanisms.

Wound healing and regeneration occur naturally in both plants and animal species. Sir William Osler (1849–1919) a physician-founder of Johns Hopkins Hospital, studied translational paradigms. He observed that some mechanisms occur ubiquitously among all living organisms (Millard 2011).

Stem cells are responsible for body mapping, growth, and organogenesis during development. Later stem cells play a role in tissue maintenance, repair and optimisation throughout an organism's lifespan (Chagastelles and Nardi, 2011). Wounding leads to a stress response that re-awakens the tissue building machinery. In plants, strategically obtained cuttings from meristem cell-rich zones such as leaves, stems and shoot tips have been used by farmers for centuries to produce phenotypically desirable crops (Jayanand *et al.* 2003). By virtue of these stem cells, tree stumps or fallen branches can regrow an entire tree. This is often done deliberately, in a process known as coppicing.

In animals, salamanders are capable of completely re-growing amputated limbs, although this process is far more elusive in mammals (Morrison *et al.* 2006). In mice with amputated digits, there is upregulation of developmental genes in order to facilitate tip regeneration (Han *et al.* 2008). However, a wounded soldier, or a patient with critical limb ischaemia, could never regenerate a limb in the same way as a tree or salamander. This is the trade-off for the complexity and intricacy of human anatomy. As a result, any damage from overuse, wear and tear, or unforeseeable circumstances cannot easily be reversed. Our carefully designed complex environment is similar.

The Second Law of Thermodynamics describes 'entropy,' or a system's propensity towards imbalance, disorder, and destruction. However, it should be noted that entropy occurs in a *closed* system. Neither the Earth, nor the human body, are closed systems. Energy exchange, inflow, and outflow between humans and the environment occurs continuously – the environment exerts an influence on humans and cyclically humans exert an influence on the environment. Despite the fact that the entropy predicts an instinct towards self-destruction, suggesting that chaos and disorder are within our nature, all living beings, both sentient and non-sentient strive for order.

Biodiversity describes the variety of organisms and habitats on Earth. This includes inter- and intra-species variety. This variety confers an evolutionary advantage through optimising adaptive capacity. Our planet is a complex ecosystem, with every structure playing a critical role. Like a food chain, disruption at one level impacts all subsequent levels. The balance and energy flow dynamic may never be restored. Extinction, ecosystem damage and the loss of biodiversity impact our lives in both predictable and unpredictable ways.

The dual use dilemma

Human relationship with the planet mirrors the relationship with individual health and body. This indicates the importance of balance. For example, food is important for sustenance but overeating leads to obesity and deterioration in health. Similarly, medications could be life-saving but over-medicating can be disastrous.

The human presence on the planet is both enriching and exploitative. This is known as a dual-use dilemma (Atlas and Dando 2006). The dual-use dilemma describes the ethical quandary that arises when actions that can be used primarily to benefit humanity can also be 'misused' in a harmful manner. For example, the environment is valued as a source of raw materials, yet humans desecrate it, using it as a sink for waste products. As a species, the human relationship with the Earth is 'parasitic', living in or on the host and benefiting by deriving nutrients, at the host's expense. On the other hand, as the most 'intelligent species,' our presence is enriching by the ability to provide order, creativity and innovation. Yet, the same qualities may make us an exploitative presence when humans use their autonomy without limits.

The dual used dilemma poses a fundamental bioethical challenge to optimise the benefit-risk profiles. 'Misuse' is a complex and controversial term to define. Knowledge is misused when it is applied in a way that is unethical or outside the scope for which it was intended. In medical history, this is seen, for example in experiments on non-consenting participants (Weindling et al. 2016). Objectively, both science and technology have improved quality of life and contributed in many ways to the evolution of healthcare and economic growth. However, overuse and unregulated use has led to abuse of these resources. Overuse has devastated the environment and, by extension, our own health.

Towards personal and planetary health: prevention and responsibility

In 2016, the WHO estimated a total of 56.9 million deaths were attributable to mostly preventable causes. The predominant cause of death was ischaemic heart disease and stroke (WHO 2020), as a result from the increasing rates of heart disease, obesity and diabetes precipitated by an ageing population. The second highest cause of death was from pulmonary conditions, including lung cancer, chronic obstructive pulmonary disorder and respiratory infections.

Despite years of effort to reduce the incidence of these conditions and numerous public health campaigns which outlining the benefits and risk of certain lifestyles, people still ignore the significance of their actions. Many individuals do not consider something important until it becomes personal to them. It could be argued that the information in public health campaigns is less effective because it is not personalised to people's lives.

In order to be effective, efforts should be focused on making people's health a priority through personalizing the message of prevention. It is highly unlikely that this will be achieved by instilling fear in the public or solely emphasizing the consequences of lifestyles, which can lead to stigma. The personalised message should encourage individuals to make healthy living a priority in their life and find realistic solutions to obstacles they face in achieving a healthy lifestyle. Prevention is the key to reversing further damage to the environment as well. But, prevention requires responsibility.

Responsibility may be distributed on two levels. The first level is investigative accountability, which identifies the person responsible for the damage. The second level of prevention is procedural accountability, which identifies the person responsible for fixing the damage. Both investigative and procedural accountability are required to close the loop of effective action.

To be sure, establishing responsibility may spark a vicious 'blame-game', which is a dangerous sport for several reasons. Firstly, when working retrospectively, it is almost impossible to obtain a complete and accurate record of the facts and processes that have led to the current state. Secondly, even if the record was complete, it would be impossible to judge this impartially. Humans are unreliable narrators of personal history and generally poor self-assessors. Thirdly, and most importantly, 'culpability' is irrelevant. Like a chronic condition, climate change is a problem that started long ago, it is multifactorial, with some of its triggers being human caused and others not. Despite these caveats, it is our responsibility to manage the problem if we wish to avoid catastrophic consequences.

Conclusion

The fate of the human race is tied to the fate of the planet. In many ways, our behaviour towards the planet mirrors our behaviour towards ourselves. Therefore, environmental ethics are a logical extension of the bioethics agenda. Regardless of who or what is to blame for climate change or personal health, the burden of responsibility now lies with us, in the present moment. The only decision that matters is the next one the human collective makes. The planet has exhausted its compensatory methods and, by extension, its capacity to self-heal. As a result, humans must pick up the mantle of responsibility, treating the planet as a sick patient and ourselves as doctors, nurturing and restoring, where possible. Thus, humankind is forced to consider the ethical, ecological, and social 'chain' of impact exerted through our actions. As a species, the ability to control ourselves and our environment is both our greatest gift and our greatest curse. Homo Sapiens are an integral part of the network of the planet's wider ecosystem. It appears counterintuitive that the most intelligent species on the planet would knowingly orchestrate the destruction of its own environment. It is this power, however that affords the capacity and responsibility to self-reflect and act ethically, using our autonomy in a manner that is beneficent, non-maleficent and just.

Disclosure statement

No potential conflict of interest was reported by the author(s).

References

Ataman, A.D., Vatanoğlu-Lutz, E.E., and Yıldırım, G., 2013. Medicine in stamps-Ignaz Semmelweis and puerperal fever. *Journal of the Turkish German gynecological association*, 14 (1), 35.

Atlas, R.M. and Dando, M. 2006. The dual-use dilemma for the life sciences: perspectives, conundrums, and global solutions. *Biosecurity and bioterrorism: biodefense strategy, practice, and science*. 4(3), 276–286.

Chagastelles PC, Nardi NB. 2011. Biology of stem cells: an overview. *Kidney international supplement* 1(3), 63–67.

Han, M., et al., 2008. Development and regeneration of the neonatal digit tip in mice. *Developmental biology* 315 (1), 125–135.

Intergovernmental Panel on Climate Change. 2001. Climate change: impact, adaptation, vulnerability [online]. Cambridge University Press, 80–115. Available at: https://www.ipcc.ch/site/assets/uploads/2018/03/WGII_TAR_full_report-2.pdf [Accessed 21 December 2019].

Jayanand, B., et al., 2003. An efficient protocol for the regeneration of whole plants of chickpea (Cicer arietinum L.) by using axillary meristem explants derived from in vitro-germinated seedlings. *In vitro cellular & developmental biology – plant*, 39 (2), 171.

Malla, A., Joober, R., and Garcia, A., 2015. 'Mental illness is like any other medical illness': a critical examination of the statement and its impact on patient care and society. *Journal of psychiatry & neuroscience*, 40 (3), 147.

Millard, M.W., 2011. Can Osler teach us about 21st-century medical ethics? *Proceedings (Bayl Univ Med Cent)*, 24 (3), 227–235.

Morrison, J.I., et al., 2006. Salamander limb regeneration involves the activation of a multipotent skeletal muscle satellite cell population. *Journal of cell biology*, 172 (3), 433–440.

Purden, A, et al., 2013. *Environmental health perspectives*. 121(8): 878–885.

Steffen, W., et al., 2015. Planetary boundaries: Guiding human development on a changing planet. *Science*, 347 (6223), 1259855.

Stewart, A.J., and Devlin, P.M., 2006. The history of the smallpox vaccine. *Journal of infection*, 52 (5), 329–334.

Weindling, P., et al., 2016. The victims of unethical human experiments and coerced research under National Socialism. *Endeavour*, 40 (1), 1–6.

Weiss, R.A., and Esparza, J., 2015. The prevention and eradication of smallpox: a commentary on Sloane (1755) 'An account of inoculation'. *philosophical transactions of the royal society of London B biological sciences*, 370 (1666), 20140378.

World Health Organization. 2020. WHO WHO Mortality Database. [online] Available at: https://www.who.int/healthinfo/mortality_data/en/ [Accessed 23, December, 2019].

Restorative Commons as an Expanded Ethical Framework for Public Health and Environmental Sustainability

ROBERT GUREVICH

Pollution is currently responsible for 16% of premature deaths worldwide and poses the greatest long-term threat to public health due to the effects of climate change. The current framework of public health cannot justify sustainability measures at an appropriate scale and timeframe to prevent further irreversible damage to the environment. To handle the issue of environmental degradation and its effect on humans, a revised framework for public health that gives more thought and consideration to the non-human environment is required. Restorative Commons theory can bridge environmental ethics and medical ethics by emphasizing the mutual benefits of environmental stewardship to nature and humans. This reflects an expansion of the environmentalist land ethic to a new 'global health ethic'. In light of this, medicine should engage with the community and the environment, in addition to treating individuals.

Introduction

Healthcare cannot ignore the significance of the environment as a factor in nearly all human illnesses, making sustainability particularly relevant to public health (Landrigan *et al.* 2017). In recent years, promising developments in healthcare sustainability that promote systems thinking include the rise of certain nature therapies, recognition of co-benefits for environmental and human health, and the shift of healthcare away from the hospital setting. Scientists, doctors, and politicians in Western countries are converging on a more holistic perspective towards healthcare. However, within the current framework of public health that is tolerant of an unjust economic system (Horton *et al.* 2014), new developments in sustainability have been and will continue to be, inadequate. To handle the issue of environmental degradation and its effect on humans, there needs to be a revised framework for public health that gives more thought and consideration to the non-human environment.

Current sustainability initiatives are limited in their scope; for example, targeted campaigns to reduce carbon footprints may achieve some measure of success, but they do not change humanity's relationship with the environment, which is the root of the issue. To more effectively handle the challenges of environmental degradation and climate change, there needs to be an expanded view of public health that gives more thought and consideration to the non-human environment.

Restorative Commons theory applied in healthcare settings can be the bridge to this new public health. Restorative Commons views the environment as a shared community space that can mutually benefit the health of humans and nature. In this light, medicine should engage with the community and the environment, in addition to treating individuals. This is a logical extension of current trends in healthcare, towards 'high-value care,' resource conservation, and alternative modes of delivery outside of the hospital setting. Certain rising forms of green therapy can complement traditional interventionist approaches and move healthcare from the view of treating individuals to a more robust global health ethic. This involves treating illness with a minimal impact on the environment, while caring for human and non-human communities in integrated green health centres. There needs to be a framework to assess health facilities based on this reconstructed relationship with nature, weighing the needs of the various stakeholders in the Restorative Commons: patient, doctor, facility, community, and environment. This is made intelligible when set within the climate crisis.

Climate crisis

The specific health consequences of climate change are extensive. For example, more frequent heat waves cause cardiovascular deaths in the elderly, particularly in urban environments. Shifting weather patterns introduce pollen into new areas, compounding with the effects of smog, especially on asthmatics. Rising global temperatures are allowing mosquitoes to populate higher-altitude mountain areas that were previously too cold. Thus, climate change results in an increased incidence of malaria by thousands of cases every year where people do not have natural immunity against malaria (Siraj *et al.* 2014). Changing water levels and droughts threaten the Caribbean seafood industry and agriculture, respectively, thus affecting people's food security. More frequent extreme weather events have been shown to increase the incidence of posttraumatic stress disorder and depression. In summary, the wide-reaching health effects of climate change are apparent, 'expected to worsen over the next century,' and thus 'must be substantially curbed' (Crowley 2016, p. 608).

The Lancet Commission calls for global action because 'pollution can no longer be viewed as an isolated environmental issue, but is a transcendent problem that affects the health and well-being of entire societies' (Landrigan *et al.* 2017, p. 464). Accepting that pollution poses an imminent threat to public health makes clear the need for sustainability across all industries, including healthcare.

Restorative Commons

The Restorative Commons theory can bridge environmental ethics and medical ethics by emphasizing the mutual benefits of environmental stewardship to nature and humans. This term was coined in 2007 at a United States Forest Service Conference highlighting practical ways to improve the health of nature and humans in a mutually beneficial way. Attended by leaders and scholars in the fields of public health, design, and resource management, the conference was meant to explore the concept of Restorative Commons as 'public space conducive to individual and community health.' The conference resulted in a report highlighting communities where urban residents' relationship to nature can have significant implications for public health (Campbell 2011).

Restorative Commons is a 'broad vision for twenty-first-century open space' where humans acknowledge their role as stewards for the environment and this creates mutual health benefits. If humans accept nature as our community, then the environment should be an inseparable part of the life course approach, because we cannot examine our lives independently of the community of which we are a part. Restorative Commons encompasses modern theories in environmental ethics that emphasize the human relationship with nature as one of the community (Campbell 2011).

The term 'commons' originally comes from the British usage, meaning unregulated public land used for purposes such as grazing livestock. It was famously introduced in the context of economics and environmental resources by American ecologist Garret Hardin in the 1968 essay 'Tragedy of the Commons.' Hardin's commons referred to any unregulated shared resource, such as land, the atmosphere, or fishing grounds. The tragedy described was that resources would be overexploited if subject to people's consciences alone, unless the public agreed to certain rules on the usage of the commons. For example, farmers would allow an unsustainable number of livestock onto shared fields to benefit themselves economically. Each farmer would act in their own self-interest, thus leading to overgrazing and harming all in the community, including themselves. Hardin concluded that the solution to the tragedy of the commons is not only technical but requires 'a fundamental extension of morality' to submit to regulations on what are currently held to be basic freedoms.

In 1999, Elinor Ostrom proved the 'Tragedy of the Commons' is not universally true in a systematic study of commons around the world. Ostrom found that if a set of conditions is met, then a community could use a shared resource in a sustainable way without top-down regulation. These conditions include: (1) clearly defined boundaries; (2) proportional equivalence between benefits and costs; (3) collective choice arrangements; (4) monitoring; (5) graduated sanctions; (6) fast and fair conflict resolution; (7) local autonomy; (8) appropriate relations with other tiers of rule-making authority (polycentric governance) (Ostrom 1999). Ten years later, Ostrom's groundbreaking work earned the Nobel Prize in Economics (Wilson 2016).

'Restorative' refers to the observed phenomenon that human health is inextricably linked to the environment. This relationship is encompassed by the theory of biophilia, the basis for many nature therapies discussed in the next section. In their introduction, the editors tie the scope of Restorative Commons to healthcare: 'How do we proceed to expand our definition of health to include the health of the land and further, to invest in the health of our landscapes as part of our healthcare programmes? What would it look like for a hospital to *steward* the land it inhabits and that of the neighbourhood it serves (Campbell 2011, p. 13, emphasis mine)?' The reference to stewardship is key to the restorative aspects of the human-nature relationship.

Restorative Commons emphasizes the role of community-based civic stewardship in the function of the urban ecosystem. Several chapters comprise case studies of infrastructure and community projects that allow urban citizens to engage with nature in a mutually beneficial way. For example, a community garden in Red Hook, Brooklyn that empowers and educates elementary school children, a horticulture rehabilitation program in prisons that reduces rates of recidivism, a New York Public Housing initiative to green the gray environment with gardens, and transforming a New York landfill into a park for the community. Restorative Commons is illustrative in theory but limited in practice because the editors do not synthesize general principles or identify challenges that may arise.

Ostrom's solution to the Tragedy of the Commons – which in the context of the atmosphere, implies total ecosystem collapse – may bridge the somewhat murky space between small-scale community projects and public health globally. By maintaining each of the eight principles, the Red Hook Community farm can run sustainably, without government regulation, based on its members' consciences alone, according to Ostrom's observations of resource-sharing communities around the world. Based on the multilevel selection, a global network of small-scale communities engaging nature sustainably will thrive due to the health benefits inherent to biophilia, while less sustainable groups will die out. The multilevel selection theory of evolution focuses on cooperation among groups, rather than competition between individuals, which was emphasized by Darwinism (Wilson 2016).

In the context of the growth of systems thinking, other groups are converging on the 'restorative' aspects of nature. The American College of Physicians (ACP) is confronting the challenge of climate change in the healthcare industry and beginning to acknowledge the environment's restorative capabilities and expanded responsibilities for physicians. 'Tackling climate change is an opportunity to dramatically improve human health and avert dire environmental outcomes, and ... ACP believes that physicians can play a role in achieving this goal ... Efforts to adapt to a changing planet and mitigate future harmful emissions could bring about major health and environmental *cobenefits* (Crowley 2016, p. 608, emphasis mine).' The cobenefits they refer to are incidental to carbon emissions reduction; for example, cycling promotes cardiovascular health and 'reducing demand for greenhouse gas-intensive meat in high-income countries' shifts people to a more healthy diet (Crowley 2016, appendix). The co-benefits perspective is a step in the right direction but is limited in scope compared to the more robust Restorative Commons view of the environment.

Significantly, the ACP does not simply defer tackling this issue to the government and outside authorities, but they recognize the responsibility of doctors and the healthcare community at large:

Physicians and the wider health care community have a major stake in addressing climate change, not only by *treating* patients experiencing its health effects but also by *advocating* for effective climate change *adaptation* and *mitigation* policies, *educating* the public about potential health dangers posed by climate change, *pushing* for a low-carbon health care sector, *researching* and *implementing* public health strategies, and *adopting* lifestyle changes that limit carbon emissions and may achieve better health. (Crowley 2016, p. 609, emphasis mine)

This expands the traditional view that a doctor's only responsibility is to the welfare of the patient. The passage above suggests a broader understanding of public health, in which concern for non-human factors is included in the best interests of the patient. While this is a bold statement for an authority as large as the ACP, their policies reflect a traditional view, which sees climate change as a pragmatic issue of damage control. Alone, their views are insufficient because they frame the environment as an opposing force that needs to be controlled – which is impossible – rather than the source of all life on Earth. A more effective approach would leverage the co-benefits aspect, and go further to view the environment with a less anthropocentric perspective.

Horton *et al.* (2014) emphasize that such a change calls for action on all levels of society. Society must mobilize and unite all efforts to control human impact on the environment. What lacks in 'Restorative Commons' is the pressing need to spread knowledge from the relatively small communities engaged in gardening and nature therapy to something that captivates the entire globe.

Ecotherapy

In recent years, healthcare has increasingly moved out of the hospital setting towards more efficient modes of delivery, some of which may be considered alternative medicine. A range of nature therapies are currently employed to treat different ailments and populations, for example, nature walks for children with attention deficits and recreational therapy for veterans with post-traumatic stress. The field of ecopsychology – of which nature therapy is a part – recognizes the health benefits of nature and seeks to apply them to various mental health problems. According to Sackett (2010), 'Ecotherapy is systemic and promotes the interconnectedness of all things. Essential to ecotherapy is the belief that healing takes place in the context of relationships, including relationships between human and nature. Nature, in and of itself is healing.' This statement is representative of a larger shift towards systems thinking in healthcare, consistent with Markevych *et al.* (2017) and Restorative Commons, recognizing the interconnectedness of nature, disease, and community, which has potential to improve health outcomes and sustainability by mutual healing.

For most of human history, until the relatively recent agricultural revolution 10,000 years ago, *homo sapiens* evolved in response to the non-human environment. As a result, we have an inherent inclination to interact with nature, a theory known as biophilia. However, since the human body and psyche developed mostly under the influence of natural, rather than anthropogenic, factors, we are still programmed to respond to a range of natural stimuli (Kellert 2016). A landmark 1986 study subliminally flashed images of spiders, snakes, frayed wires, and handguns to subjects and found the natural threats elicited a negative response, while the human stimuli usually caused no reaction (Ohman 1986). These findings show that we retain an emotional response to the natural environment; however, this adaptation is likely to atrophy over time as it becomes vestigial.

There is a large body of evidence supporting the link between nature and human health. Improved mental health, reduced obesity, higher birth weights, improved mortality, and improved child behavioural development have been linked to greenspace exposure among urban residents (Markevych *et al.* 2017). The Markevych study found three specific pathways to health through nature. Nature may assist health by reducing harm, restoring capacities, or building capacities.

Markevych's three pathways of ecotherapy

The reducing harm pathways focus on avoiding the health effects of anthropogenic climate degradation. The latter are well documented, extensive, and disparate – ranging from more frequent heat waves causing thousands of cardiovascular-related deaths among the elderly (Crowley 2016) – to the effect of increased air-particulate matter on osteoporosis (Prada *et al.* 2017). Other harm reduction pathways are as follows: less exposure to air pollutants in greenspace,[1] cooler temperatures due to mitigation of the urban heat island effect, and lower perceived noise, which has many psychological implications. Pollution, heat and noise have each been shown to correlate with poor health outcomes.

The related restorative and building pathways mediate nature and health. Restorative pathways examine nature's capacity for psychological and physiological restoration. This may encompass stress reduction theory (SRT) and attention restoration theory (ART), which each responds to antecedent conditions affecting health created by the nonhuman built environment. In modern society, our habitat has become chiefly a constructed world. While the shift away from bio-centric interaction with the environment to electronic media has revolutionized our society, there have also been specific negative effects on health. Children engage with electronic media more than fifty hours each week on average, but play outside for less than seven hours each week (Kellert 2016).

Stress reduction theory holds that exposure to greenspace rapidly promotes a positive emotional state that mitigates the body's stress response to the built environment. Physiological measures including blood pressure as well as psychological measures, such as self-reported emotional state before and after nature walk support this theory (Ulrich *et al.* 1991). More experimentation needs to be done to determine the specific mechanisms by which nature mitigates the stress response, as well as the effect of different levels of exposure, e.g. the setting (park, forest, garden) and duration.

Attention restoration theory, on the other hand, is concerned with the ability of nature to reduce attention fatigue by holding a person's attention without effort,

---

[1] Which is not to say that greenspace reduces air pollutants overall, rather, there is evidence to the contrary (Markevych et al. 2017).

'thereby enabling rest of the neurocognitive mechanism on which effortful directed attention depends' (Markevych *et al.* 2017). Markevych *et al.* note the difficulty of making attributions to either SRT or ART since stress often has an effect on attention and vice versa. However, both theories are still useful in explaining the restorative effects of the natural environment.

Finally, the 'building' capacities of nature encourage physical activity and facilitate social cohesion. Greenspace provides an attractive setting for exercise and exercise in green areas can, in turn, have greater psychological and physiological benefits than exercise indoors. However, greenspace and developed land use for exercise must be balanced because a preponderance of undeveloped land results in increased car dependency (Markevych *et al.* 2017). Green areas are also significant as community spaces that facilitate social cohesion within neighbourhoods, which has been shown to have a significant positive effect on mental and general health (Dadvand *et al.* 2017). Even though the three pathways are meant to mediate the effect of greenspace exposure on the health of urban residents, they also provide a useful framework for understanding the mechanisms behind nature therapy, especially where other explanations are lacking.

Significantly, scientists are not the only ones converging on the 'restorative' capabilities of nature. Restorative Commons emphasizes the same restorative and community potential as the three pathways but from the perspectives of environmentalism and agriculture.[2]

Ecotherapy and veterans

While the therapeutic value of recreation is well documented, the particular benefits of recreation in nature for veterans with war injuries have only been studied recently (Hawkins *et al.* 2016). Veterans of modern wars are returning with similar sets of injuries and the health system of the Department of Veterans Affairs (VA) has been inadequate in treating them. Veterans have frequently complicated cases with multiple factors; 49% of soldiers returning from war screen positive for polytrauma. Posttraumatic stress (PTS) and traumatic brain injury (TBI) have been called signature injuries of the 'War on Terror' and are the most common facets of polytrauma (Hawkins *et al.* 2016). Current treatment options offered by the VA are cognitive behavioural therapy to confront the triggers of PTS and antidepressants such as selective serotonin reuptake inhibitors (SSRIs), which can have severe side effects. These treatment modalities reflect a deficits approach to healthcare. Moreover, there is a stigma that prevents many veterans from seeking psychiatric care or makes them averse to taking medication for their polytrauma. In addition to proper treatment from military trauma, ultimately, society should seek to reduce wars, not only because of the effects on people, but also the effect on nature, ecosystems, and the significant carbon footprint of defense (Bailey 2009).

Veterans are increasingly turning to outside organizations for eco- and recreational therapies, which leverage a 'strengths-based approach' specifically tailored to their needs (Hawkins *et al.* 2016). These therapies emphasize their internal and external strengths, as well as existing military skillsets, to create an empowering

---

[2] However, Restorative Commons and the three pathways are limited in scope by their focus on high-income countries.

experience through various nature-based interventions, including outdoor adventure therapy, wilderness therapy, and outdoor experiential therapy. Nature settings are well suited to a strengths-based approach because the environments used are inherently more supportive than traditional healthcare settings. The therapies typically involve taking small groups on several-day expeditions emphasizing physical skills, such as climbing, hiking, or fly-fishing, and do not overtly involve psychiatric 'treatment,' rather they foster camaraderie and discussion among veterans about their experiences.

Common features of these therapies are (1) novel settings where the veterans are unsure of themselves; (2) perceived risk forcing them to confront their fears; and (3) small groups that require interdependence. Hawkins *et al.* (2016) compared these therapies to traditional treatments and their 'results indicated statistically significant decreases in negative mood states, depression, anxiety, PTS symptoms, somatic symptoms of stress and perceptual stress, as well as improvements in attentiveness, positive mood states, and sleep quality (p. 65).' However, Hawkins *et al.* did not address the sex of their participants. Sex will need to be addressed in ecotherapy moving forward, given that female veterans have a 63% higher incidence of PTS (Xue *et al.* 2015).

The use of ecotherapy and veterans confirms Markevych's framework linking greenspace and health since nature induced a state of 'calm alertness' (Hawkins *et al.* 2016, p. 65), rather than the disconcerted alertness many veterans experience. In this reduced stress environment, veterans restored the attention fatigue resulting from their polytrauma and experienced many health benefits.

Concretely, the government should consider giving the VA resources to fund nature recreation therapy as an appropriate treatment for polytrauma. Nature therapy can treat a range of illnesses as a complement to traditional medical practice and promotes the Restorative Commons. While additional research needs to be done on the field of nature therapy, its potential as a sustainable medical treatment is clear.

Health centres and sustainability

Until recently, the healthcare field was slow to adapt to environmental changes because it was evaluated based on traditional bioethics, with the patient and doctor as the only stakeholders. Traditional medical ethics tells us that sustainability should not be a primary concern in patient care. In ethics and practice, the first tenet is 'do no harm,' and as such, most efforts are directed toward the welfare of the patient.

Sustainability in traditional health care centres
Medical ethics conventionally address patient autonomy and dilemmas arising from new treatment methods and technologies (Beauchamp and Childress 2001). To focus on sustainability can be seen as diverting resources, not least of which is a physician's time and attention, from the patient. Some believe that policies of sustainability are in violation of patient autonomy and therefore unethical. Consider

the effective cancer drug Taxol, which once made from large quantities of the endangered Pacific Yew tree (Jameton and McGuire 2002, p. 121). People affected by cancer might say, 'To hell with the trees,' and seek the latest treatment at any cost.

One underlying reason for such blatant disregard for sustainability in medicine is the narrative of nature being the 'enemy' (Jameton and McGuire 2002, p. 118). Examples of this include the 'War on Cancer' initiative started by former U.S. President Nixon, as well as hospitals struggling to contain antibiotic-resistant 'superbugs.' This ethical balance opposing biology versus human well-being is a moral hazard that makes it paradoxical to seek to preserve nature.

Another predominant normative theory, Virginia Held's *Ethics of Care* (2006), focuses on caring relationships as opposed to medical duties. If a doctor's interpretation of care ethics is limited to relationships between people, then she has the right to say, 'This is just not part of my job,' when asked to consider the environment.

Lastly, there is an economic argument against sustainability. Medicine is already very costly to patients and the government and investing into sustainability would further increase their financial burden. To offer 'eco-friendly' medical treatments as an optional public-relations booster would naturally lead to these becoming a premium option, similar to organic foods. This creates a second moral hazard that precludes economically disadvantaged patients from sustainability, even though they are more likely to be harmed by climate change and need medical services. Thus, a traditional argument is that to be democratic and keep prices down, the healthcare business must not offer sustainable treatment options.

Sustainability in green health care centres

In response to these traditional rebuttals, the reasons for integrating the environment, bioethics and healthcare are threefold: (1) The threat of climate change is real and requires immediate action. (2) The healthcare industry causes significant pollution that can be reduced without any consequences at the bedside. (3) Environmental design principles can be applied successfully to healthcare, albeit requiring a reevaluation of some ethics principles pertaining to dilemmas that arise with traditional bioethics. These dilemmas must first be resolved before moving forward with planning sustainable healthcare practices and infrastructure.

The traditional normative frameworks outlined above lack the foresight to improve, or even maintain, the current standard of medical care for future generations. Eckelman and Sherman (2016) report that healthcare is one of the leading polluting industries in the United States, as a result of energy use and emissions from hospitals and manufacturing, particularly. This causes environmental degradation such as poor air and water quality. The resulting health impact, in terms of total years of patient life lost per year, is comparable to the annual deaths resulting from medical error in the United States (Eckelman and Sherman 2016). Therefore, the first step to sustainable healthcare is to recognize that the current pattern of increasing resource and energy use, as well as waste production, causes serious damage to the biosphere and human health. Further, if we do not take deliberate social action to control pollution, the resulting damage to the environment will be irreversible and our ancestors will have to deal with serious health consequences (Jameton and McGuire 2002).

Sustainability is not a priority in U.S. healthcare even though the industry's harmful environmental effects are well documented. In 2013, healthcare was one of the leading contributors to pollution in the United States, 'including acid rain (12%), greenhouse gas emissions (10%), smog formation (10%),' all of which affect public health (Eckelman and Sherman 2016). Despite these facts, medical ethics remains principally concerned with questions of patient care. Healthcare businesses look out for a number of other stakeholders, but the environment is largely ignored.

Case study in a green health care centre

Once other stakeholders are introduced, the environment becomes a significant concern. The Universities of Nebraska and Florida provide practical examples of integrating sustainability into modern health-care centres that embody Restorative Commons. The University of Nebraska Medical Center (UNMC) was one of the first to undertake a comprehensive campus-wide sustainability initiative, known as the Green Health Center. Andrew Jameton and Catherine McGuire, lead bioethicists for the project, summarize its goals as follows:

> The provision of health care for present generations must not undermine the ability of ecosystems to support future generations. Health care practice must reinforce the restoration and maintenance of global ecosystems. And, the clinical and environmental activities of health care must be conducted with fairness and without exploitation. (2002, p. 116)

The UNMC recognizes that the results of not enforcing environmental stewardship (e.g. causing cancer) directly contradict the principle of 'do no harm'.

In order to 'link bedside concerns to the larger context of global environmental well-being' (Jameton and Pierce 2001, p. 366), UNMC regards sustainability for the purpose of healthcare as having three concerns: patient, economy, and environment (Jameton and McGuire 2002, p. 114–115). Using this modified 'triple bottom-line' can refute the above arguments against sustainability.

To suggest that sustainability initiatives contradict the principle of 'do no harm' erroneously assumes that they sacrifice some aspects of patient welfare. Yet this flat-out ignores the health implications of pollution. However, making healthcare production more economical does not affect patient care. The UNMC purchases supplies from companies that consider their upstream effects, e.g. the sourcing of latex for gloves. UNMC also plans its transportation routes for lower emissions. Hospital air conditioning systems are a major source of energy use that can be made more efficient while remaining 'behind-the-scenes' of patient care (Hermes 2014).

Further, it is possible to reduce and reuse supplies while maintaining the standard of care – for example, expensive single-use surgical instruments can be sterilized and used several times without a significant increase in infection rate (Hermes 2014). Being mindful of waste can reduce emissions as well. Anything deemed biological waste is usually incinerated; however, many wastes, such as used supplies, can be sterilized and landfilled or recycled, rather than burned. All of these methods maintain the patient as the top priority, while being economical and eco-friendly.

Another facility which has successfully moved toward being a Green Medical Center is the University of Florida. Frumkin traces the history of green construction in healthcare, starting with the University of Florida, which has set aside 300 acres, or 15%, of their campus as a nature preserve free for patients, students and visitors to enjoy (2007). With approximately 50,000 students, a stadium and many buildings, the University is essentially a city a within a city, owning the utilities, waste treatment, and transport infrastructure; as such, they are committed to using their resources sustainably.

Since 2001, all new construction at UFL has been LEED certified. The University has accumulated a significant portion of all such buildings in the entire state. In some areas, they have gone beyond the LEED standards, with more efficient toilets, preserving trees on campus, local sourcing of construction materials, and committing to green power in some buildings. These steps have further reduced the environmental footprint. This is more than just a perfunctory political move to be 'green'; the UFL has seen a cultural shift towards sustainability and integrated it into medical education in its various medical facilities. This has improved the patient experience and shown to be economical for the hospital (Frumkin 2007).

Jameton claims medical knowledge is part of the 'commons'; physicians do not own it. This view 'expresses a strong articulation of a stewardship model' (Pierce and Jameton 2004, p. 88). Therefore, conservation of resources that benefits the most people is a natural extension of a doctor's professional responsibilities. Environmental implications are inherent to evidence-based medicine; however, such decision-making still requires special training and institutional backing. Ultimately, doctors are not at liberty to make decisions based on environmental concerns alone, thus they need institutional support. This further strengthens the argument that sustainability must be integrated from a top-down approach, via the policy of a Green Health Center. When resources are controlled, this does not disenfranchise the patient with fewer options but empowers them to make more meaningful choices.

Assessment methods for Restorative Commons in health care

Once the ethical foundations are solid, sustainability and nature must be considered in a Green Medical Center from its very construction. This must be done empirically and scientifically, the same standards for any other developments in healthcare. Measuring performance in light of this expanded framework for public health requires an equally nuanced assessment system. Since healthcare is full of standards, assessments, ratings, and checklists, it would be appropriate to devise such a scheme in light of Restorative Commons. Quantifying waste, practicing the '3 R's' – reduce, reuse, recycle – energy efficiency, and integrative building design are metrics of Restorative Commons.

Quantify waste

Frumkin (2007, p. 5) claims 'Simply claiming that something *is green*, without demonstrating empirical benefits for health and well-being, the environment, and economics is not enough.' Towards this end, the issues of waste and recycling are of particular concern for the medical field. An observation piece in the *Scientific American* blog identifies unique recycling obstacles faced by science laboratories that account for their surprising lack of sustainability (McCoy 2017). Many university medical centres are also hubs for research, which are a major contributor to the site's overall waste output. For instance, the labs of McGill University generate 100 tons of plastic waste and 250 tons of glass every year; the US alone has more than 300 research universities. Single-use products such as latex gloves, test tubes, and pipettes comprise much of this waste. They are necessarily autoclaved to sanitize them and then landfilled. Switching over to reusable versions of these products is possible, albeit inconvenient, compared to individually packaged, single-use supplies.

Reduce, reuse, recycle

To counteract the allure of single-use supplies, McCoy suggests incentivizing reusing and recycling on a government or lab level, reducing the total waste output. There are instances of similar programmes having some measure of success, such as Emory University having a separate grant line for sustainability-related projects. Another possible strategy would be to penalize recyclables found with the regular waste (McCoy 2017). The strategies McCoy suggests could be applied to healthcare because of the common issues with single-use supplies and sterilization. This would ensure healthcare contributes to public health, rather than landfills.

Energy efficiency

Since healthcare facilities now consume twice the average amount of energy for commercial buildings, the need for efficiency is paramount. The federal government developed Leadership in Energy and Environmental Design (LEED) to provide a benchmark for the construction of new green facilities with the following goals:

> [To promote] the practice of (1) increasing the efficiency with which buildings and their sites use energy, water, and materials, and (2) reducing building impacts on human health and the environment through better siting, design, construction, operation, maintenance, and removal— the complete building life cycle. (US Green Building Council, in Frumkin 2007, p. 10)

LEED guidelines take a comprehensive, whole-building approach focusing on the areas of sustainable site development, energy efficiency, water savings, materials, and indoor environmental quality. Healthcare presents unique challenges to green construction due to the high energy use – which stems mainly from air conditioning – and maintaining a healthy indoor environment, resulting in a very low proportion of LEED projects in the sector. In 2004, only 2% of LEED buildings were health facilities. However, as constructors overcome the learning curve, the cost premium – now typically in the range of 1–3% for a LEED building – is shrinking every year and offset by savings on energy. Further, when a company has one LEED building, they are more likely to adhere to the guidelines on future construction (Frumkin 2007).

Integrative building design

Beyond efficiency, a green health centre should integrate nature in a way that promotes health. The presence of windows with natural views in recovery rooms has been shown to dramatically reduce the length of hospital stays and improve psychological state (Ulrich 1984). Nature must be integrated into site design with a big picture approach since biophilia holds we are evolutionarily inclined to thrive in it. Site planning is particularly important to maximize daylight exposure. Bringing natural materials and scenery into interior spaces improves patients and staff perception of the hospital environment (Frumkin 2007). Frumkin shows not only the benefits of sustainability for hospitals but also the potential of healthcare to promote the notion of planetary health and a global health ethic. Since a hospital's mission is improving the welfare of the populace, the construction and appearance of a medical facility should communicate the same message.

With increasing attention to the issue of climate change, progressively sophisticated assessments are being created, such as LEED Healthcare, which evolves sometimes on a weekly basis, making compliance difficult for administrators and constructors. However, hospitals favour check-lists, and there is no shortage of sustainability check-lists being developed, often with complex hierarchies weighing different environmental factors and subfactors (Aljaberi et al. 2017). Adapting these to healthcare would require consideration of the Restorative Commons.

To this end, some existing systems show promise and can be used as the basis for new ones. Many are along the lines of LEED applied to built structure, but lack depth in considering the other aspects of sustainability such as user-friendliness, health outcomes, and management issues. These systems sometimes have modular additions for healthcare construction, as in the cases of LEED and the British BREEAM (Castro et al. 2015), however, they are all limited in scope to building infrastructure. Evaluation systems specific to healthcare, such as the widespread Joint Commission International accreditation system, started in the US in 1994, are focused with a standard of care and efficiency, but not sustainability. Given its widespread use, a Joint Commission accreditation ensures the same standard of care between hospitals in different countries that employ it (Buffoli et al. 2015).

Summary

Currently, the Public Health literature lacks an assessment system where the environment, patient care, and operational factors are all considered on the same scale. In light of Restorative Commons, where environmental health is an integral factor of public health, there needs to be a new evaluation system combining the advantages of environmental health and public health, augmenting medical care issues with sustainability as part of a robust package, rather than the environment being an ancillary factor.

A successful assessment system would mirror this centralized approach, such as those found at the Universities of Nebraska and Florida, where sustainability is integrated into operations in a comprehensive manner as part of the organizations' mission, and consider the various stakeholders in healthcare – patient, doctor, community, business, environment. The weight to give each of these stakeholders is a challenge demanding close, multidisciplinary consideration.

Once in place, this system can be the basis for ensuring conformity with Restorative Commons and government penalties for violators. Sustainability, when enacted, is self-perpetuating. After the initial investment into infrastructure, sustainability is quite efficient. Conserving energy, reducing waste, and smarter use of supplies could save $15 billion over 10 years, according to the Commonwealth Fund (Hermes 2014). Regulations making sustainability the industry standard would eliminate the moral hazard of making sustainable healthcare seem like a premium option, like organic food. This would be superior to the currently vague, non-committal statements governments make in favour of environmental sustainability, such as the Paris Accords.

Conclusion

Early conservationist and environmental ethicist Aldo Leopold wrote about humanity's relationship with the environment as one of the community as early as the 1940s. Goldberg and Patz (2015) expand Leopold's 'land ethic' to a 'global health ethic' as a logical way to guide society in recognizing the importance of our place in the environment – the mutual relationship between planetary and human health. Perhaps Restorative Commons is the link between a land ethic and a global health ethic, a way to attract society's collective attention to the significance of the environment. Make no mistake, we must change our outlook on sustainability quickly in order to effectively address climate change in an appropriate timescale. The future of humanity is at stake.

Disclosure statement

No potential conflict of interest was reported by the author(s).

References

Aljaberi, O.A., Hussain, M., and Drake, P.R., 2017. A framework for measuring sustainability in healthcare systems. *International journal of healthcare management*, 1–10. doi:10.1080/20479700.2017.1404710.

Bailey, J.J., 2009. Is it practical for defence to reduce its carbon emissions without affecting its effectiveness? *Defence studies*, 9, 47–84.

Beauchamp, T.L., and Childress, J.F., 2001. *Principles of biomedical ethics*. 5th ed. New York: Oxford University Press.

Buffoli, M., et al., 2015. Healthcare sustainability evaluation systems. *In*: S. Capolongo et al., eds. *Improving sustainability during hospital design and operation*. Cham: Springer, 23–29. Available from: htps://link.springer.com/chapter/10.1007/978-3-319-14036-0_3.

Campbell, L., 2011. *Restorative commons*. Revised ed. Newtown Square, PA: USDA Forest Service.

Castro, M., Mateus, R., and Bragança, L., 2015. A critical analysis of building sustainability assessment methods for healthcare buildings. *Environment, development, and sustainability*, 17, doi:10.1007/s10668-014-9611-0.

Crowley, R., 2016. Climate change and health: a position paper of the American College of Physicians. *Annals of internal medicine*, 164, doi:10.7326/M15-2766.

Dadvand, P., *et al.*, 2017. Lifelong residential exposure to green space and attention: a population-based prospective study. *Environmental health perspectives*, 125, doi:10.1289/EHP694.

Eckelman, M.J., and Sherman, J., 2016. Environmental impacts of the U.S. health care system and effects on public health. *Plos one*, 11, doi:10.1371/journal.pone.0157014.

Frumkin, H., 2007. *Green healthcare institutions: health, environment, and economics. Institute of medicine*, doi:10.17226/11878.

Goldberg, T., and Patz, J., 2015. The need for a global health ethic. *The lancet*, 386, doi:10.1016/S0140-6736(15)60757-7.

Hawkins, B., *et al.*, 2016. Nature-based recreational therapy for military service members: a strengths approach. *Therapeutic recreation journal*, 50, doi:10.18666/TRJ-2016-V50-I1-6793.

Held, V., 2006. *The ethics of care: personal, political, and global*. Oxford: Oxford University Press.

Hermes, J. 2014. Minimizing environmental footprint while delivering affordable healthcare. Available from: http://www.environmentalleader.com/2014/11/minimizing-environmental-footprint-while-delivering-affordable-healthcare/.

Horton, R., *et al.*, 2014. From public to planetary health: a manifesto. *The lancet*, 383, doi:10.1016/S0140-6736(14)60409-8.

Jameton, A., and Pierce, J., 2001. Environment and health: sustainable health care and emerging ethical responsibilities. *Canadian medical association journal*, 164, 365–369.

Jameton, A., and McGuire, C., 2002. Toward sustainable healthcare services: principles, challenges, and a process. *International journal of sustainability in higher education*, 3, 113–127.

Kellert, S.R., 2016. Nature in buildings and health design. *In*: J. Barton *et al.*, eds. *Green exercise*. London: Routledge Ltd, 17–25. doi:10.4324/9781315750941.

Landrigan, P.J., *et al.*, 2017. The Lancet commission on pollution and health. *The lancet*, 391, doi:10.1016/S0140-6736(17)32345-0.

Markevych, I., *et al.*, 2017. Exploring pathways linking greenspace to health: theoretical and methodological guidance. *Environmental research*, 158, 301–317. doi:10.1016/j.envres.2017.06.028.

McCoy, K. 2017. Why are scientists so bad at recycling? Scientific American blog. Available from: https://blogs.scientificamerican.com/observations/why-are-scientists-so-bad-at-recycling/.

Ohman, A., 1986. Face the beast and fear the face: animal and social fears as prototypes for evolutionary analyses of emotion. *Psychophysiology*, 23, 123–145. doi:10.1111/j.1469-8986.1986.tb00608.x.

Ostrom, E., 1999. Coping with tragedies of the commons. *Annual review of political science*, 2, 493–535.

Pierce, J., and Jameton, A., 2004. *The ethics of environmentally responsible health care*. Oxford [u.a.]: Oxford Univ. Press.

Prada, D., *et al.*, 2017. Association of air particulate pollution with bone loss over time and bone fracture risk: Analysis of data from two independent studies. *The Lancet planetary health*, 1, doi:10.1016/S2542-5196(17)30136-5.

Sackett, C.R., 2010. Ecotherapy: a counter to society's unhealthy trend? *Journal of creativity in mental health*, 5, 134–141. doi:10.1080/15401383.2010.485082.

Siraj, A.S., *et al.*, 2014. Altitudinal changes in malaria incidence in highlands of Ethiopia and Colombia. *Science*, 343, 1154–1158. doi:10.1126/science.1244325.

Ulrich, R.S., 1984. View through a window may influence recovery from surgery. *Science*, 224, doi:10.1126/science.6143402.

Ulrich, R.S., *et al.*, 1991. Stress recovery during exposure to natural and urban environments. *Journal of environmental psychology*, 11, doi:10.1016/S0272-4944(05)80184-7.

Wilson, D. 2016. The tragedy of the commons: how Elinor Ostrom solved one of life's greatest dilemmas. Available from: http://evonomics.com/tragedy-of-the-commons-elinor-ostrom/.

Xue, C., *et al.*, 2015. A meta-analysis of risk factors for combat-related PTSD among military personnel and veterans. *PLos One*, 10, doi:10.1371/journal.pone.0120270.

Part II
Ethical Practice for Environmentally Sustainable Health Care

The Climate Emergency: Are the Doctors who take Non-violent Direct Action to Raise Public Awareness Radical Activists, Rightminded Professionals, or Reluctant Whistleblowers?

Terry Kemple

When doctors become aware of a threat to public health, they have a professional duty to try to mitigate the threat. Climate change is a recognized major threat to planetary and public health that requires actions to both mitigate, and adapt to, climate change. The limited time and resources available to change what humankind are doing and protect planetary health add urgency to the threat. Some doctors take non-violent direct actions if their governments fail to take the effective actions needed. Professional regulatory organizations like the UK's General Medical Council (GMC) are charged with protecting the health of patients by setting standards for, giving ethical advice about, and supervising the behaviour of doctors. This article examines the conflict between climate activist doctors and the GMC interpretation of a doctor's duty of care when there is threat to public health from climate change.

David Roberts recently remarked, 'For five decades now, [climate models] have warned us that we are marching toward ruin, and we have, for the most part, ignored them. We cannot claim that we did not know what we were doing' (2019). Humankind is waking up to the consequences of living unsustainably. Medicine mostly uses the lens of its discipline to zoom in on the most specialized studies of the human body or zoom out to get the bigger picture in public health. Yet, if physicians want to help people to stay healthy, the lens must zoom out beyond public health to view the health of the planet and try to understand and manage its complex natural systems. Planetary health links the disruptions of the Earth's natural systems caused by humans with the resulting impacts on public health and then develops and evaluates evidence-based solutions to maintain a world that is healthy and sustainable for everyone. Anticipating and avoiding futures that can cause worse public health should be possible from understanding threats like climate change and reacting fast enough by switching away from environmentally damaging ways of living to sustainable ways.

The extra challenge of climate change for humankind is that there is limited time and resources to change what is being done and protect planetary health. Most governments (UNFCC 2015) have acknowledged the problem of climate change and made pledges to mitigate it but there is a widespread consensus that not enough is being done; governments are failing to fulfil their existing pledges to take the necessary actions (Carbon Brief 2019).

As public awareness of the enormity of the threats to planetary health increases, social movements like Extinction Rebellion (XR), which demand urgent action, are growing. These movements may include non-violent direct actions as part of their protests. This article examines the ethical dilemma for doctors in the UK who consider climate change a major threat to public health threat and take non-violent direct actions to raise awareness and influence government but then come into conflict with the government and its professional regulator of doctors in the UK – the General Medical Council.

Ethical foundations: the Golden rule or Kant's categorical imperative

The principle of treating others as you want to be treated yourself is a common, but not universal, maxim of reciprocity. As a moral duty if it is accepted, it becomes the foundation for other often-cited advice about human interactions. The principle is widespread – in philosophy it is recognized in Kant's categorical imperative (Kant and Paton 2009) and in religion and culture it is often known as the Golden rule. In this article, the concept will be referred to as the Golden rule. The variations in the application of the Golden rule are how humans can reasonably expect to be treated by all others, and how much humans can extend these expectations to others. The latter may be applicable to those who are distant in place and time, such as inhabitants of far off countries and the future unborn generations.

Society's expectation for acceptable behaviours can react with the issues of the time so humans must be prepared to change how they interpret and adhere to the Golden rule. For example: those who were brought up in a Roman Catholic household in the UK in the mid-twentieth century were expected to follow the rules described in a pocket-sized book called the 'Catechism.' This was also known as the Penny Catechism. It provided the elementary structure of the Catholic Faith for generations of people until the 1960s. Catholic children were given this small book to study in the early years at school. The catechism included the Jewish 'Ten

Commandments' and other doctrines of the Catholic church. Children learned about the so-called 'Golden rule'.

Today's version of the small pocket-sized catechism, *The Catechism of the Catholic Church* (Catechism of the Catholic Church 2019). was introduced in the 1990s. It is an oversize book with 900+ pages. It is still changing. In November 2019, following through on a proposal made at the Synod of Bishops for the Amazon, Pope Francis said there are plans to include a definition of ecological sins in the church's official teaching. 'We should be introducing – we were thinking – in the Catechism of the Catholic Church the sin against ecology, ecological sin against the common home' (Catholicnews.com 2019). This language of ecological sin was unthinkable a century ago, or even a decade ago.

Currently, the awareness and acceptance of the threat from climate change and its impact on the planet varies among people. Most individuals need to be more aware about the threats to health on the planet and then act to reduce the risks of climate change. However, learning and accepting the essential information about climate change and then the next steps of appropriately changing behaviours, either as well-informed citizens or dutiful doctors, does not always occur. The reactions to climate change can include a call to action, but also denial, environmental grief, climate depression, eco-anxiety, futilitarianism, or becoming a 'doomer'. This different awareness, and then acceptance of, these threats and impacts by individuals and organizations inevitably cause problems applying the Golden rule consistently. The interval between becoming aware of a threat and taking action can undermine the efficacy of the Golden rule.

If the outcome of a rule does not work out as expected, thoughtful people should ask the question whether it was conceptual failure or implementation failure. There are only trivial reasons to believe the Golden rule is flawed and the concept wrong, thus eliminating conceptual failure. The poor outcome of the Golden rule must be an implementation failure; humans have been unable to deliver on our self-chosen principles.

The problem of implementation of the Golden rule

Falsehood flies and the truth comes limping after it. Jonathan Swift (1710)

There are many different explanations for the human behaviour responsible for implementation failure of the Golden rule. Once each is identified, perhaps they can be mitigated. These explanations include mechanisms like the following and are applicable to individuals and organizations like the General Medical Council (GMC).

First, there are the familiar processes of normal and accepted psychological reactions. For example, the adaptive behaviour that humans can feel around experiences like loss and grief. The stages of this process include shock and denial, pain and guilt, anger and bargaining, depression and reflection. All are common in the context of personal reactions about climate changes.

Second, are the less familiar cognitive phenomena of heuristics and biases described by Kahneman (2011). Individuals cope with uncertainty and complexity by using a small number of general-purpose heuristics for simplifying judgments and making decisions. This can lead to suboptimal decision-making.

Third, humans, as individuals, follow a unique mix of rules rooted in personal truths, deceits, biases from upbringing, family mores, religious rules, the dominant culture, generational norms and the laws of the land. Professions like medicine add another set of rules. These can all be influenced by false rules and fake news, for example, the mistaken belief that repetition is a form of validation. The character of the Bellman by Lewis Carroll in 'The Hunting of the Snark' says 'What I tell you three times is true' (1876). This Bellman-like deceit is apparent in scientific research in the continued presentation of discredited data, or the disregard of data from a study which comes to a different conclusion. A modern example is the antivaxxer belief that autism is caused by the Mumps, Measles and Rubella (MMR) combined immunization in childhood. Despite subsequent retraction by the publishing journal of the fraudulent research that started this false finding, the paper is still widely cited and believed (Suelzer *et al.* 2019). The Bellman-like deceit is a common and widely applied mistake, perhaps because humans often look either for confirmation of an existing bias, or are disinclined to challenge the false information.

Fourth, in addition to conscious biases, humans also have unconscious biases. Self-Tests can measure implicit attitudes and beliefs and reveal unconscious bias. These Implicit Association Tests (Greenwald *et al.* 1998) are widely available on-line and usually reveal a bias that people are either unwilling or unable to report.

Fifth, the outcomes of all these psychological processes, heuristics, rules and biases make us who we are and manifests through phenomena like conscience, 'common sense' and 'gut reactions'. Conscience can warn that something is wrong, or suggest that something is right. Expert intuition in any profession is a specialized gut reaction recognition of patterns. The individual expert may not be consciously aware that something that does not fit in the expected pattern, but the mind can process information more quickly than one can comprehend it (Reason 2009). There is a great danger in leaping to the wrong conclusions when there is insufficient information. This creates the 'strong but wrong' reaction in the mind.

Given these and other obstacles, a few strategies can mitigate the implementation failure of the Golden rule. Individuals and organizations can learn to recognize and ignore many of the obstacles to implementation. Individuals can expect to get wiser if they can learn from their mistakes. Although it may be not be possible to discover any great truth, it is possible to recognize mistakes earlier and more often. The opposite of wisdom is the stupidity of making the same mistake over and over. Only the wisest and stupidest never change.

The ethical codes given to doctors

Ethical codes are given to doctors at graduation from their medical school and after graduation from medical organizations. Doctors refer to these codes throughout their practice and use them to protect and defend them from those outside of the profession. Many are based in a deontological ethics, which reflects the Golden rule.

Initial secular pledges at graduation

Many medical schools expect their student to take an oath or pledge at their graduation. This has its origins in the earliest expression of medical ethics in the western world: the Hippocratic oath (Edelstein 1943). In 1948, the World Medical Association (WMA) was concerned over the state of medical ethics and drafted a pledge – the Declaration of Geneva (wma.net 1948) – so that the oath's moral code could be passed on in a modern way. In the 1960s, the Hippocratic Oath itself was changed to make it a more contemporary and secular obligation (Lasagna 1964).

There are various versions of these pledges and there are always pressures to update their contents. For example, in many countries campaigns to allow legal assisted-dying is a common call for change in the pledges. There is also pressure from doctors concerned about planetary health to require 'protection of the environment which sustains us' and extend the focus of care for doctors from the individual to the community and the ecosystem. In 2008, Dr Margaret Chan, the director of the World Health Organisation stated, 'in the face of this challenge, the WHO is committed to do everything it can to ensure all is done to protect human health from climate change' (Chan 2008).

Continuing national professional regulators and influencers after graduation

In addition to, or in the absence of, oaths and pledges upon their qualification, doctors are expected to follow the rules of their national professional regulatory authority that each publish, and police their versions of the rights and responsibilities – the duties – of a doctor. In the UK, the General Medical Council provides a comprehensive overview of the obligations and professional behaviour of a doctor to their patients and wider society (gmc-uk.org 2013). Doctors who violate these codes may be subjected to disciplinary proceedings, including the loss of their licence to practice medicine (gmc-uk.org 2020a). The General Medical council was created by an Act of Parliament in 1858 entitled 'An Act to Regulate the Qualifications of Practitioners in Medicine and Surgery' (Legislation.gov.uk 1858). It was the first to regulate the practice of doctors in the UK.

At its start, the General Medical Council was a body of doctors who self-regulated their profession. This model allowed doctors themselves to decide what was best for patients. Its disciplinary powers were exercised only in cases of criminal behaviour or poor professional conduct for the time, often summarized as the '3 A's': addiction, adultery and advertising. Modern regulations are less rigid about some of these conducts. Scandals regarding patient safety, and some disquiet that the organization was self-serving, prompted the reform of the GMC into an independent regulator (legislation.gov.uk 1978).

The GMC published the first edition of its *Good Medical Practice* (gmc-uk.org 2013) in 1995. This gave the first explicit statements about the standards of care patients should expect and doctors should provide. Although the original self-regulated GMC was an inadequate safeguard for patients, its successor – the independent regulator GMC – is not safe from censure.

High-quality organizations usually have robust governance that allows a constant process of feedback to challenge and improve practice. There may be guardians in charge of the rules and their interpretation in an organization, but there should not be anonymous rule makers and enforcers who cannot be challenged. There should be identifiable people with roles. The British politician Tony Benn suggested that you should be able to search out the named people in charge and then ask: 'What power have you got? Where did you get it from? In whose interests do you exercise it? To whom are you accountable? And how can we get rid of you?' (Benn 2001). Organizations with insufficient feedback, quality improvement, and assurance in the processes of regulation can preserve flawed processes and outcomes.

The GMC has an implicit duty to take appropriate actions to identify and reduce the risks when there are threats to the public's health. The GMC already accepts and follows its public duty and holds financial investments only through fund managers who demonstrate the strongest environmental, social and governance credentials and specifically excludes investment in companies that derive more than 10% of their revenue from: tobacco, alcohol, gambling, pornography, high-interest rate lending, cluster munitions and landmines, and the extraction of thermal coal or oil sands (Gmc-uk.org 2018a). Whilst more and more medical organizations are divesting from energy companies that rely on fossil fuels and investing in companies generating energy from renewable sources, the GMC continues to permit its own investments in the fossil fuel industry.

The GMC has declared, 'doctors in particular have a duty to act when they believe patients' safety is at risk, or that patients' care or dignity are being compromised.' (gmc-uk.org 2013). Doctors themselves have a professional duty to report themselves to the GMC when they are charged with, or found guilty of, a criminal offence. The GMC then usually refers the doctor to a medical practitioner's publicly held tribunal that conducts an investigation and makes a judgement. Some specific and less serious convictions like parking and speeding offences do not have to be referred for investigation (gmc-uk.org 2020b). Although speeding has a known association with risks of harm to other people it has not been recognized as an important offence, perhaps because it is a highly prevalent offence.

If the tribunal judges that a doctor's fitness to practise is impaired, it has a few options. First, it can take no action. Second it can agree to undertakings offered by the doctor at the hearing. Third, it can put conditions on the doctor's registration, which restricts what a doctor is allowed to do. Fourth, it can stop a doctor from working as a doctor for a set period of time (suspension). Fifth, it can remove the doctor from the medical register to stop them practising (erasure) (mpts-uk.org 2020). Regardless of the final outcome, the tribunal process is usually slow, long, and stressful for the doctor who is being investigated and judged.

Other softer, but important, influencers in professional behaviour are the predetermined performance pathways, such as guidelines, and payments for performance that are used to attempt to link various aspects of doctors' work, including effort, achievement, values, purpose, and self-understanding, to measures and comparisons of output and outcomes.

All these regulations and guidelines can be like satellite navigation on car journeys: authoritative and useful, but prone to major errors at difficult junctions. Although they can seem obligatory, they are in reality just informed advice and not a guarantee of the best outcome.

The ethical codes used by doctors

The secular pledges and professional regulations usually set only the basic and minimally acceptable standards for doctors. Importantly, there are other sets of standards that also apply. Integrity, moral duty and quality are words that can express the nature and importance of these higher standards. Doctors learn these higher standards through lifelong learning experiences. Humans are influenced by many things, including the Golden rule itself, positive and negative roles models, peer group pressure, the breadth and depth of personal experience, and feedback from others. All knowledge is formed by information with experience, context, interpretation, and reflection.

Professional judgement, like any practical wisdom, is a form of knowledge that is not formally taught, but is acquired through experience. Explicit knowledge for physicians typically uses the evidence-base of medicine. Tacit knowledge however is based on personal know-how. Greater wisdom can develop through continuing critical deliberation about the best thing to do in practice. This is more than learning from simple reflection.

In medicine, wisdom is the use of a clinician's professional judgement that helps individuals manage the uncertainties and risk in their lives. Professional judgement is important when doctors decide not to follow published guidelines for care. A dilemma of modern health care is that doctors are trained and expected to use their judgement for the best interests of their patients, but well-intentioned prescriptive regulations and guidelines may hinder them from using their best judgement.

Many doctors continue to aspire to higher standards to provide 'quality' care for their patients. 'Quality' often describes a specific vagueness in performance in medicine and it is not always clear what quality means for most people. Lewis Carroll's Humpty Dumpty 'understood' the words he used. 'When I use a word, it means just what I choose it to mean – neither more nor less' (Carroll 1871). Quality, like many concepts, is often used without a shared understanding and it will frequently mean different things to different people at different times.

Quality may often describe more of a journey of aspiration for greater achievement with milestones on the way rather than a fixed destination or accomplishment. The problem with the quality journey is that, although there is a direction to take, the final destination may change. Quality is a higher aspiration than even the Golden rule – to treat others even better than you expect to be treated yourself. When doctors treat other doctors they often try to provide the highest of standards, because if they themselves become patients, they often expect the highest of standards.

There are informal and formal accreditation systems for quality standards in most countries. Although self-assessment of quality can often be considered an inadequate safeguard of minimum standards, the state-regulated quality assessments can become bureaucratic obstructions to quality improvement and learning by promoting caution and conformity. To assure quality the GMC introduced the mandatory relicensing of doctors every 5 years, through a process called revalidation and a list of requirements that aim to reduce unacceptable variations in the care by doctors. Regulators can set arbitrary and inappropriate standards and may have little tolerance for contrary ideas or opinions. The list of requirements can become more valued than the purpose of the process.

Adherents to any dogma run the risk of increasing their efforts to obey, and unwillingness to change the rules and thereby risk undermining the Golden rule. The desired outcome of quality assurance becomes a casualty of the bureaucracy. Such may be the case when physicians are obligated to act only on guidance that is broadcast from the top down, rather than mastered from the bottom up.

Physician activism

The UK's General Medical Council tells doctors that they do have a duty 'to act when they believe patients' safety is at risk' (gmc-uk.org 2013). The GMC also assures them they will be protected if they follow a process that results in their whistleblowing (gmc-uk.org 2018c). Doctors who believe climate change is the major threat to the health of the majority of people on the planet may become frustrated that governments and other responsible organizations like the GMC are not responding sufficiently to mitigate the threat. Any non-violent actions that doctors may take to raise awareness can conflict with the laws of the land and the rulings of the national regulators of doctors who determine the standards of care that patients should expect and the behaviour that doctors should follow.

Despite their duty to act and the GMC's assurance of support, if doctors attempt to raise awareness about the threat of climate change and the government's failure to mitigate climate change, i.e. 'whistleblow' and then get arrested after taking non-violent actions, they make themselves liable to be disciplined for unprofessional conduct by the GMC and labelled as radical activists by the popular media.

For example, in April 2019 Dr Diana Warner was one of six people in the original 'Extinction Rebellion' (XR) movement who staged a protest on a train at a London station by using a super glue to attach herself to a train window. She was arrested and charged under the Malicious Damage Act of 1861 but a scheduled Crown court jury trial in May 2020 was postponed due to the Covid-19 pandemic. Following the outcome of the court appearance she would await a judgement about her behaviour by the GMC (Mahase 2019).

Doctors for Extinction Rebellion

Extinction Rebellion was started in the UK in May 2018, but it quickly became an influential environmental mass movement. With the stated aim to be a global movement that uses non-violent civil disobedience in an attempt to halt mass extinction and minimize the risk of social collapse, XR has three demands: First, tell the truth. Governments must tell the truth by declaring a climate and ecological emergency, working with other institutions to communicate the urgency for change.

Second, act now. Governments must act now to halt biodiversity loss and reduce greenhouse gas emissions to net zero by 2025. Third, go beyond politics. Governments must create and be led by the decisions of a Citizens' Assembly on climate and ecological justice (Extinction Rebellion 2018).

Extinction Rebellion has explicit principles and values, but the organization is decentralized, meaning that there is no requirement for each local XR group to ask for permission from a central group or authority. Arguably, this has helped it to be both a faster growing, and faster learning, organization.

In May 2019, a new special interest XR group called 'Doctors for Extinction Rebellion' (Mahase 2019) formed in the UK to fight climate change and promote planetary and public health. Many doctors who are concerned about their government's failure to acknowledge the climate emergency and failure to defend life are taking part in non-violent direct action, such as demonstrations that occasionally result in arrests for offences such as obstruction of a police officer, breach of the public order act, breach of the peace, obstruction of the highway, aggravated trespassing, criminal damage and theft, violent disorder, and affray. These arrests are often used by police to clear away a demonstration and those arrested are subsequently released without any charge or criminal record. Any arrests of physicians that result in being charged with a crime, or being convicted, can trigger referral by the GMC to the Medical Practitioners Tribunal Service. The Tribunal will make an investigation and give a public hearing. These protestors may be viewed in different ways – as radical activists, right-minded professionals, or reluctant whistleblowers.

Radical activists?

In an ideal world, scientists would report on science and the government would act on it. Unfortunately, this has not happened with climate change. So, to get this critical message out, some doctors are resorting to civil disruption to get in the press and inform the public to pressure government to act on the science.

Dr Chris Newman, a General Practitioner and a co-founder of Doctors for Extinction Rebellion remarks,

> there is a deep sense that we as healthcare professionals must become advocates for the ecosystem as a vital part of health, and that to do this most effectively we must step out of our traditional roles. We are held in high regard by the public, and we must honour their faith by acting in a manner that matches the magnitude of the problem. (Mahase 2019)

If, in the course of these non-violent direct actions, doctors are arrested, charged and appear in the courts, they can then use that platform to further raise awareness of the major threats to public health. Although this has been shown to be effective, these doctors are often dismissed as radical activists by naysayers and the media.

Labelling others with false descriptors by 'name calling' that which society generally deems negative, alienates the activists and discredits their message. It can create a strong – but wrong – reaction to them and their message. When this does happen, reframing the problem can make it easier to understand and interpret. To change thought processes, awareness of the current framing must be developed, consequences considered, an alternative frame devised, and the consequences of alternative innovative thinking considered.

In challenging the description of Extinction Rebellion as a radical environmentalist movement, Scott Fraser reframed the argument: 'Extinction Rebellion has rightly sought to bring to wider attention the imminent breakdown of our climate and the catastrophe this will herald if we do not change our behaviour very soon. I can't see how this would be described as radical: we don't label smoking cessation practitioners as 'radical anti-cancers' or school crossing patrols as 'radical anti-accident activists' (Fraser 2019).

Right minded professionals doing their duty?

The climate emergency is like no other in recorded history. Dr Chris Newman, questions,

> why do we spend billions of pounds every year reducing small—yet statistically significant—(health) risks to small groups of people, yet spend so little on unimaginable risks to everyone? What happens when our duty to safeguard public health directly conflicts with the authority of government? (Mahase 2019)

Dr Newman called on the General Medical Council to support doctors taking direct action against climate change and was himself was one of several doctors who was arrested after scaling and then gluing themselves to a government building in London in September 2019. They carried out the act of 'peaceful civil disobedience' to deliver an 'urgent health warning' about the severity of the climate and ecological crisis, and to prompt government action on the matter (Iacobucci 2019). Newman explained

> climate and ecological breakdown pose one of the greatest threats to public health the world has ever faced. Yet the government is failing to take meaningful steps to protect its citizens. Non-violent peaceful protests like today are essential public health interventions for getting the government to take immediate action.

Following the code of self-reporting, Newman wrote to the GMC after his arrest and urged the UK's regulator to declare a climate and environmental emergency and support doctors taking action, stating,

> We do still expect you to hold doctors to account for their actions as part of protest groups, but if and only if they are deemed to be wholly excessive. There should be no 'carte blanche' for protestors, but fear of giving this does not justify the prolonged delay thus far in making your climate declaration.

In a statement related to doctors who protest about climate change the GMC responded, 'like all citizens, doctors are entitled to their own political opinions, and there is nothing in the standards that we set that prevents them from exercising their rights to lobby government or campaign' (Iacobucci 2019). By this statement the GMC seems to muddle the scientific facts about the threats to health from climate change with political opinions about what governments should do.

The GMC went on to write:

> If we were to receive a complaint or a self-referral about the actions of a doctor involved in a protest, we would have a legal duty to consider the matter raised. However, as with all complaints, we would make our decision based on the specific facts of the case. Our focus would be on whether the doctor's actions may have fallen seriously or persistently below the standards we set or put patients or the public confidence in the profession at risk. Doctors must always be prepared to justify their decisions and actions.

The GMC added: 'We understand the strength of the concerns that doctors are raising about the impact of climate change. However, our role is set out in the Medical Act, which provides us with no powers to declare a climate emergency' (Iacobucci 2019).

Climate change will affect most people and may cause a great transformation all over the world. What should any right-minded doctors do when they become aware of the threat to human health from climate change and the need to mitigate and adapt to climate change? Each person should consider their moral duty informed by the Golden rule, then follow their own conscience.

Reluctant whistleblowers?

Quis custodiet ipsos custodes?' (Translation: 'Who will guard the guards themselves'?) is generally used to consider the embodiment of the philosophical question as to how those in power can be held to account. Although the GMC may view physicians who take non-violent direct actions as political activists, perhaps a more useful way to view physician activism – including those who take non-violent direct actions – is that of whistleblowers doing their professional duty. In doing so, doctors may be following the Golden rule and prompting others, including the GMC, to do the same and change their behaviour.

According to the GMC, 'whistleblowing' is where an employee, former employee or member of an organization raises concerns to people who have the power and presumed willingness to take corrective action' (gmc-uk.org 2018c). A broader definition might recognize that a whistleblower is usually someone who exposes information or activity that is deemed illegal, unethical or incorrect within a private or public organization. Discussions on whistleblowing usually consider attempts to define whistleblowing more precisely, with debates about whether and when whistleblowing is permissible, and debates about whether and when one has an obligation to blow the whistle.

In the UK, whistleblowers are protected by law and should not be treated unfairly because of whistleblowing. The law specifically protects whistleblowers who report that someone's health and safety is in danger, report risk or actual damage to the environment, or report if someone is suspected of covering up wrongdoing. Anna Rowland, the Assistant Director of Policy, Business Transformation and Safeguarding GMC claims, 'we want whistleblowers to feel confident in raising their concerns to us and so we have improved the process by which disclosures can be made, giving people the option to do so anonymously' (gmc-uk.org 2018b).

It is in the best interests of the public for physicians to safeguard the future of patients' health by speaking out about the damaging consequences to public health of climate change. A physician who raises awareness about climate change and threats to health, and exposes the lack of sufficient actions by government and other organizations, including the GMC, to mitigate climate change seems to be acting – knowingly or unknowingly – as a whistleblower. Whistleblowers risk reprisal and retaliation from those who are accused or alleged of wrongdoing. Doctors can be concerned that the General Medical Council does not acknowledge the whistleblowing nature of their actions and does not protect them.

Rita Issa, a co-founder of Doctors for Extinction Rebellion remarks,

> as a doctor, I'm bound by good clinical practice to hold human life with the utmost respect, to practise from a scientific evidence base, and to act promptly when patient safety may be compromised ... and I'm supporting Extinction Rebellion ... out of duty to this ethical code, and out of respect to the evidence that the climate crisis is, as the Lancet called it, 'the greatest threat to human health of the 21st century. (Moberly 2019)

The GMC has a duty to support whistleblowers, even when the GMC is the organization being accused of the wrongdoing.

Conclusion

The GMC, and UK Government, should acknowledge the grave threat to the environment and public health of climate change and take appropriate actions to identify and reduce threats to public health. The concept of the Golden rule and its implementation are a measure of the quality of health care. Medical pledges, regulatory authorities and Government policies should be aligned to support the actions of doctors attempting to implement the Golden rule. When this alignment is missing, then the quality assurance of health care may be failing, and the root causes of that failure should be sought. Being open to feedback – including whistleblowing – is essential to correct misalignments and the ability to tackle urgent issues like climate change.

Disclosure statement

No potential conflict of interest was reported by the author(s).

References

Benn, T. 2001. *House of commons hansard debates for 22 Mar 2001 (pt 13)*. [online]. Publications.parliament.uk. Available from: https://publications.parliament.uk/pa/cm200001/cmhansrd/vo010322/debtext/10322-13.htm [Accessed 3 March 2020].

Carbon Brief. 2019. *COP25: Key outcomes agreed at the UN climate talks in Madrid | Carbon Brief* [online]. Available from: https://www.carbonbrief.org/cop25-key-outcomes-agreed-at-the-un-climate-talks-in-madrid [Accessed 3 March 2020].

Carroll, L., 1871. *Through the looking-glass*. London: MacMillan.

———., 1876. *The hunting of the snark*. London: Macmillan Publishers.

Catechism of the Catholic Church. 2019. Vatican City: Libreria Editrice Vaticana.

Catholicnews.com. 2019. *Catechism will be updated to include ecological sins, pope says* [online]. Available from: https://www.catholicnews.com/services/englishnews/2019/catechism-will-be-updated-to-include-ecological-sins-pope-says.cfm [Accessed 3 March 2020].

Chan, M., 2008. *WHO | Message from WHO Director-General* [online] Who.int. Available from: https://www.who.int/world-health-day/dg_message/en/ [Accessed 3 March 2020]

Edelstein, L., 1943. *The hippocratic oath, text, translation and interpretation*. Baltimore: Johns Hopkins Press.

Extinction Rebellion. (2018). *Our demands – extinction rebellion* [online] Available from: https://rebellion.earth/the-truth/demands/ [Accessed 3 March 2020].

Fraser, S., 2019. Extinction rebellion: who is the BMJ calling radical environmentalists? *BMJ*, 365, l2256.

Gmc-uk.org. 2013. *Good medical practice* [online]. Available from: https://www.gmc-uk.org/ethical-guidance/ethical-guidance-for-doctors/good-medical-practice [Accessed 3 March 2020].

———.. 2018a. *Annual report* [online]. Available from: https://www.gmc-uk.org/-/media/documents/annual-report-2018-english_pdf-80413921.pdf [Accessed 3 March 2020].

———.. 2018b. First regulators whistleblowing report published [online]. Available from: https://www.gmc-uk.org/news/news-archive/first-regulators-whistleblowing-report-published [Accessed 3 March 2020].

———.. 2018c. *GMC policy on whistleblowing* [online]. Available from: https://www.gmc-uk.org/-/media/documents/DC5900_Whistleblowing_guidance.pdf_57107304.pdf [Accessed 3 March 2020].

———.. 2020a. *Reasons for licence withdrawal* [online]. Available from: https://www.gmc-uk.org/registration-and-licensing/managing-your-registration/revalidation/revalidation-resources/revalidation-licence-to-practise-withdrawing-giving-up-restoring-appeals/reasons-for-licence-withdrawal [Accessed 3 March 2020].

———.. 2020b. *Referral for a hearing at the MPTS* [online]. Available from: https://www.gmc-uk.org/concerns/information-for-doctors-under-investigation/our-sanctions/referral-for-a-hearing-at-the-mpts [Accessed 3 March 2020].

Greenwald, A., McGhee, D., and Schwartz, J., 1998. Measuring individual differences in implicit cognition: The implicit Association Test. *Journal of personality and social psychology*, 74, 1464–1480.

Iacobucci, G. 2019. Campaign group urges GMC to support doctors taking direct action against climate change. *The BMJ* [online]. Available from: https://www.bmj.com/content/366/bmj.l5785/related [Accessed 3 March 2020].

Kahneman, D., 2011. *Thinking, fast and slow*. New York: Farrar, Strauss and Giroux.

Kant, I., and Paton, H., 2009. *Groundwork of the metaphysic of morals*. New York: Harper Perennial Modern Thought.

Lasagna, L. 1964. NOVA *doctors' diaries, the hippocratic oath: modern version* PBS [online]. Pbs.org. Available from: https://www.pbs.org/wgbh/nova/doctors/oath_modern.html [Accessed 3 March. 2020].

Legislation.gov.uk. 1858. *Medical Act 1858* [online]. Available from: http://www.legislation.gov.uk/ukpga/Vict/21-22/90/enacted [Accessed 3 Mar. 2020].

———.. 1978. *The Medical Act 1978 (Commencement No.4) Order 1980* [online] Available from: http://www.legislation.gov.uk/uksi/1980/1524/made [Accessed 3 March 2020].

Mahase, E., 2019. Doctors for Extinction Rebellion: new group fights for planetary and public health. *BMJ*, 365, l2364.

Moberly, T., 2019. Doctors join Extinction Rebellion demonstrations. *BMJ*, 367, l6037.

Mpts-uk.org. 2020. *Overview of medical practitioners tribunal hearings and the MPTS* [online]. Available from: https://www.mpts-uk.org/-/media/mpts-documents/part-1—resource-for-doctors-medical-practitioners-tribunals_pdf-76540670.pdf?la=en&hash=A359EE761368837FC8AE38746771783B30FE1742 [Accessed 3 Mar. 2020].

Reason, J., 2009. *The human contribution: unsafe acts, accidents and heroic recoveries.* Farnham: Ashgate Publishing Ltd.

Roberts, D. 2019. *Scientists have gotten predictions of global warming right since the 1970s* [online] Vox. Available from: https://www.vox.com/energy-and-environment/2019/12/4/20991315/climate-change-prediction-models-accurate [Accessed 3 March 2020].

Suelzer, E., *et al.*, 2019. Assessment of citations of the retracted article by Wakefield et al with fraudulent claims of an association between vaccination and autism. *JAMA network open*, 2 (11), e1915552.

Swift, J. 1710. *The Examiner*, (14).

Unfccc.int. 2015. *Paris agreement* [online]. Available from: https://unfccc.int/files/meetings/paris_nov_2015/application/pdf/paris_agreement_english_.pdf [Accessed 3 March 2020].

Wma.net. (1948). *WMA – The World Medical Association-Declaration of Geneva* [online]. Available from: https://www.wma.net/what-we-do/medical-ethics/declaration-of-geneva/ [Accessed 3 March 2020].

Will the Plant-Based movement Redefine Physicians' Understanding of Chronic Disease?

Maximilian Andreas Storz

The world is experiencing a cataclysmically increasing burden from chronic illnesses. Chronic diseases are on the advance worldwide and treatment strategies to counter this development are dominated by symptom control and polypharmacy. Thus, chronic conditions are often considered irreversible, implying a slow progression of disease that can only be hampered but not stopped. The current plant-based movement is attempting to alter this way of thinking. Applying a nutrition-first approach, the ultimate goal is either disease remission or reversal. Hereby, ethical questions arise as to whether physicians' current understanding of chronic illness is outdated and morally reprehensible. In this case, physicians may need to recommend plant-based diets to every patient suffering from chronic conditions, while determining what other socio-ecological factors and environmental aspects play a role in the chronic disease process. This article provides insights to aspects of diet and chronic illness and discusses how the plant-based movement could redefine current understanding of chronic disease. The ethical justifications for recommending of a plant-based diet are analyzed. The article concludes that not advocating for plant-based nutrition is unethical and harms the planet and patients alike.

Introduction

The world is experiencing a cataclysmically increasing burden from chronic illness (Hajat and Stein 2018). Cardiovascular disease, obesity, diabetes and other chronic conditions spread around the globe like an unstoppable virus. The number of patients suffering from multiple concomitant lifestyle-related conditions is skyrocketing – without any prospect of sustained improvement. According to Hajat and Stein (2018), current data suggest that up to 57% of adults in developed countries suffer from more than one chronic condition. In 2020, 157 million Americans are expected to live with at least one chronic condition and the future health care work-force is not projected to include an appropriate mix of personnel capable to deal with this trend in a multidisciplinary manner (Bodenheimer *et al.* 2009).

From an economical perspective, this alarming development imposes a growing burden on insurers, government health programmes, and businesses (Barnard 2013). At present, more than 85% of health care costs are attributable to chronic health conditions in the United States (Beckman 2019). The rising epidemic of diabetes and obesity is now outstripping most preventive efforts, adding further to the cost of healthcare and costing lives (Williams 2017).

From an ecological point of view, current trends are appalling and lead into a virtual *cul-de-sac*. The healthcare sector, and hospitals in particular, is a major contributor to worldwide carbon emissions (McGain and Naylor 2014, Tomson 2015, Pichler *et al.* 2019). Increasing patient numbers suffering from chronic lifestyle-related disease will inevitably result in additional medical interventions and procedures which, in turn, will further contribute to a steadily rising hazardous waste production, energy expenditure and, finally, depletion of natural resources.

Treatment approaches for chronic conditions, such as cardiovascular disease, rheumatoid arthritis and diabetes, are often dominated by symptom control and risk factor management. This is, *inter alia*, the result of our current understanding of the terms 'chronic disease' and 'chronic condition'. Although definitions appear inhomogeneous and vary tremendously in the academic literature (Bernell and Howard 2016), most include some common features.

Chronic illnesses are usually prolonged, difficult to treat (Bell *et al.* 2016) and do not resolve spontaneously. They are rarely completely cured, require ongoing medical attention and 'limit activities of daily living' (Warshaw 2006). Moreover, chronic conditions are associated with impairment or disability (Bell *et al.* 2016) and have a detrimental influence on a patient's quality of life (Whittemore and Dixon 2008, Somrongthong *et al.* 2016). In short, many definitions imply the basic idea of a generally slow progression of disease that can only be hampered, but not stopped.

The current plant-based movement is attempting to fundamentally alter this way of thinking. By practicing a nutrition-first approach (Ha 2019), participating healthcare professionals aim for a different path. While classical polypharmacy-dominated treatments often target temporary relief of symptoms, the nutrition-first approach is based on a diametrically opposed understanding of chronic conditions. Instead of a mere management of symptoms and slowing down disease progression, the ultimate goal is disease reversal, which means remission of clinical symptoms and normalization of relevant laboratory values. To understand this concept, a closer look at the plant-based movement and vegan eating patterns is required.

Plant-based nutrition and vegan diets

The proportion of individuals deciding to follow a vegan diet has significantly increased within recent years (Radnitz *et al.* 2015). Within the plant-based movement, unhealthy nutrition is considered the key factor for the development of several chronic conditions such as obesity, diabetes and cardiovascular disorders. According to Kahleova *et al.* (2017), almost one half of cardio-metabolic deaths in the United States could be prevented through proper nutrition.

The consumption of a Western diet, including large amounts of red meat, poultry, fish, dairy products and eggs is seen as the common denominator promoting inflammatory reactions (Zinöcker and Lindseth 2018), diminished endothelial function (Esselstyn 2017), insulin resistance (McMacken and Shah 2017) and immunogenic compounds such as N-Glycolylneuraminic acid (Neu5Gc) in the human body (Tangvoranuntakul *et al.* 2003). It has been often suggested that a Western diet rich in animal foods leads to increased inflammation, reduced control of infection, increased risk for allergic and auto-inflammatory disease and even increased rates of cancer (Myles 2014).

Plant-based diets avoid or heavily restrict the frequency of animal food consumption (Satija and Hu 2018). According to Ostfeld, a plant-based diet excludes all animal products, including red meat, fish, poultry, eggs, and also dairy (2017). Instead of animal products, a whole-food, plant-based diet emphasizes vegetables, legumes, fruits, whole grains, nuts, herbs and seeds. Due to the frequent intake of fruits, vegetables, whole grains, and legumes, a plant-based diet is high in fibre and rich in vitamins and minerals (Physicians Committee for Responsible Medicine 2019). Since animal products are usually excluded, it is also free of cholesterol, and low in calories and saturated fat (Coulston 1999).

It should be taken into account that the term *plant-based* is sometimes used interchangeably with *vegan* or *vegetarian* (Tuso *et al.* 2013). Technically, however, this is not correct since a vegan (or total vegetarian) diet on the one hand stringently excludes all animal products (meat, seafood, poultry, eggs, and dairy products), while it does not require consumption of whole foods or restriction of fat and refined sugar on the other. Vegetarian diets exclude meat and fish consumption but may include dairy products (lacto-vegetarian) or eggs (ovo-vegetarian) (Timko *et al.* 2012, Patelakis *et al.* 2019)

Unhealthful vegan diets including large amounts of less-healthy and processed plant foods (sweetened beverages, refined grains, fries and sweets) were associated with an increased risk for coronary heart disease (Satija *et al.* 2017). Therefore, caloric intake still requires attention and patients need to be taught that foods that are labelled vegan are not necessarily healthful because they are often dense in calories and high in sodium (Radnitz *et al.* 2015). Vegan diets adopted for religious or ethical reasons may or may not be healthy, heavily depending on what kind of foods they include and not only on what they exclude (Tuso *et al.* 2013). Therefore, it seems prudent to emphasize eating healthy, and whole, plant-based foods while avoiding or heavily restricting the frequency of animal food consumption.

Patients are subsequently encouraged to refrain from refined and (ultra) processed foods (Tuso *et al.* 2013), including savoury snacks, reconstituted meat products and substitutes, pre-prepared frozen dishes, and soft drinks (Lawrence and Baker 2019). While usually free from animal-suffering, popular meat substitutes for example are often rich in sodium, emulsifiers, monosodium glutamate, flavours, colours and other cosmetic additives. A higher consumption of such ultra-processed foods (>4 servings daily) was independently associated with a 62% relatively increased hazard for all-cause mortality (Rico-Campà et al. 2019). Of note, benefits from consuming a plant-based diet will be relative to the level of frequency, as well as the amount, of animal products consumed (Tuso et al. 2013). As a corollary, emphasizing a healthy diet requires physicians not only to encourage patients to refrain from animal product consumption, but also to stress the importance of whole, plant-based foods.

It is of paramount importance that more and more societies and academies recommend the use of vegetarian and vegan diets. In a 2016 position paper, the Academy of Nutrition and Dietetics recognized vegan diets appropriate for all stages of the life cycle, including childhood, adolescence, pregnancy, lactation, infancy, older adulthood and also for athletes (Melina et al. 2016). Another renowned organization, the British Dietetic Association, recently affirmed that a well-planned vegan diet can support healthy living in people of all ages (British Dietetic Association 2020).

The use of a plant-based diet as a means of prevention and treatment has frequently been shown in both clinical and epidemiological studies. These findings could slowly but steadily lead to a new understanding of chronic conditions.

Disease reversal

A whole-food plant-based diet is the key to understand disease reversal (Klaper 2019). A diet that strictly excludes animal products may not only stop the progression of many chronic conditions, but has the potential to reverse them. The most prominent example of this is cardiovascular disease.

Cardiovascular disease

Heart disease remains the single largest cause of death in countries of all income groups (Nowbar et al. 2019). Despite more than 40 years of aggressive drug and surgical interventions (Esselstyn et al. 2014), cardiovascular disease is also the leading cause of loss of disability-adjusted life years globally (Stewart et al. 2017). Millions of patients around the globe suffer from angina – an impairing condition that is often just temporarily relieved by pharmacological treatment.

Dean Ornish and colleagues demonstrated that a plant-based diet – combined with a lifestyle programme including moderate aerobic exercise – may substantially help affected patients (1998). According to the results of their randomized trial, patients that received the described lifestyle intervention for one year reported a remarkable 91% reduction in angina attacks. The control group in this study included patients that were asked to listen to the advice of their physicians. Astonishingly, these patients had a 186% increase in reported attack frequency. The long-term effects in regard to chest pain frequency and severity were comparable to that of coronary artery bypass surgery or angioplasty (Greger 2015). Lifestyle interventions are cheaper and do not bear the side effects of surgical procedures or pharmacological treatments.

Of note, other subsequent studies that focused primarily on adoption of a plant-based diet without additional exercise revealed comparable results. A landmark study by Esselstyn and colleagues included 198 patients with significant coronary artery disease (Esselstyn *et al.* 2014). The subjects in this study suffered from multiple comorbidities such as hyperlipidaemia ($n = 161$), hypertension ($n = 60$), and diabetes ($n = 23$).

The patients were prescribed a whole-food plant-based diet, including whole grains, legumes, lentils, other vegetables, and fruits. Added oils and processed foods that contain fish, meat, fowl and dairy products were not allowed. During the following four years of follow-up, angina improved significantly in approximately 93% of patients. Moreover, 99.4% of the participants who followed the plant-based diet avoided any major cardiac event – including myocardial infarction – stroke and death. Unfortunately, 21 participants did not adhere to the prescribed diet and more than 60% (13/21 participants) of them consecutively experienced an adverse event.

In a more recent editorial, Esselstyn (2017) compared the findings from his trial to other well-known studies including the COURAGE trial (Boden *et al.* 2007) and the Lyon Diet Heart Study (de Lorgeril *et al.* 1999), which both consisted of conventionally treated participants. The author concluded that there is more than a 30-fold positive difference in major cardiovascular events when individuals eat a whole food plant-based diet (Esselstyn 2017). Findings from Esselstyn *et al.* (2014) strongly suggest that dietary change is the most active ingredient (Greger 2015) in reducing cardiovascular events. Plant-based diets are not only capable of slowing progression of coronary artery disease, but can reverse it. In many cases, this is possible without medication and additional procedures (Massera *et al.* 2015, Mejia *et al.* 2016).

It is now widely accepted that diets higher in plant foods and lower in animal foods are associated with a lower risk of cardiovascular mortality and morbidity (Kim *et al.* 2019). The fact that plant-based nutrition has beneficial effects on several established cardiovascular risk factors, such as hypertension (Alexander *et al.* 2017), adds to the overwhelming body of evidence. A meta-analysis by Yokoyama *et al.* (2014a) revealed that consumption of vegetarian diet was associated with lower mean systolic blood pressure (- 6.9 mmHg; 95% CI, −9.1 to −4.7; $p < .001$) and diastolic blood pressure (−4.7 mmHg; 95% CI, −6.3 to −3.1; $P < .001$) in comparison with the consumption of a conventional diet.

Disease reversal by adopting a plant-based diet has been observed in various other chronic conditions affecting millions of people worldwide. Another example frequently cited in the literature is type 2 diabetes.

Type 2 diabetes

Type 2 Diabetes has been referred to as the 'Black Death' of the twenty-first century in terms of its detrimental economic impact and devastating health burden (Matthews and Matthews 2011). Since the 1980s, the global prevalence of diabetes has nearly quadrupled (NCD Risk Factor Collaboration 2016) and the costs of the disease and its consequences will substantially increase by 2030 (Bommer *et al.* 2018). This development is most alarming, considering the fact that the disease is caused mainly by poor diet and lifestyle habits (Barnard 2013).

Findings from large epidemiological cohort studies several years ago revealed that a low fat, plant-based diet is associated with a substantial and independent reduction in diabetes incidence (Tonstad *et al.* 2013, Satija *et al.* 2016). In a series of clinical trials, the American physician Neal Barnard and his team of researchers and physicians consistently demonstrated the effectiveness of a vegan diet in individuals suffering from type 2 diabetes.

In 2003, Barnard and colleagues performed one of the first major randomized clinical trials in in the field. Subjects with type 2 diabetes were told to consume a purely plant-based (vegan) diet. The latter was compared to a conventional diet based on the 2003 American Diabetes Association (ADA) guidelines. After only 22 weeks, haemoglobin A1c fell 1.23 points in the vegan group, compared to 0.38 points in the control group ($p = 0.01$). Furthermore, a substantial decrease in body weight was observed (−6.5 kg in the vegan group and 3.1 kg in the ADA group ($P < 0.001$)). The same cohort was followed for a total of 74 weeks, showing a significant absolute reduction in haemoglobin A1c of −0.40 points in the vegan group versus +0.01 in the ADA group. Dr. Barnard repeatedly presents such cases during conference lectures and in his books (2007).

The effectiveness of a plant-based, vegan, diet in patients suffering from type 2 diabetes has also been shown by a meta-analysis by Yokoyama and colleagues (2014b). A plant-based diet is a powerful tool – not only for preventing and managing type 2 diabetes – but also for reversal of clinical symptoms (Davis *et al.* 2019, McGoey-Smith *et al.* 2019). It is crucial to note that a disease that was once associated with steadily progression can take a completely different course. Adoption of a plant-based diet may lead to remission of clinical diabetes symptoms and normalization of relevant laboratory values, such as glycated haemoglobin (HbA1c). The latter is an important and commonly used indicator of long-term glycaemic control, reflecting the cumulative glycaemic history of the preceding three months in patients suffering from type 2 diabetes (Sherwani *et al.* 2016, Pan *et al.* 2019).

Diabetic neuropathy

One of the most prevalent complications of diabetes is diabetic neuropathy (Feldman *et al.* 2019). The disease, which has a lifetime prevalence of approximately 50% (Juster-Switlyk and Smith 2016), is often resistant to conventional treatment. According to Greger (2015), the disease is one of the most frustrating clinical conditions to treat. Patients often respond insufficiently to pharmacological treatment and suffer from both marked impairment in daily activities and a significantly reduced quality of life.

Considering these findings, it is even more remarkable that a simple lifestyle intervention, including a vegan, plant-based diet, can actually lead to complete remission of clinical symptoms (Greger 2015). The rapid regression of neuropathic pain after initiation of lifestyle changes was reported more than two decades ago (Crane and Sample 1994). Patients suffering from diabetes and concomitant moderate or worse systemic distal polyneuropathy were enrolled in this trial. Subjects were prescribed a low fat vegan diet, which was high in fibre and unrefined foods. In addition to that, the 25-day in-residence life-style programme included daily conditioning exercise.

Complete relief of the neuropathic pain occurred in 17 of the 21 patients within just 4–16 days. Of note, the 17 responders were followed for another period of 1–4 years. In all but 1 of the 17 patients, the relief from the systemic distal polyneuropathy had continued, or there was further improvement.

A newer study by Bunner et al. (2015) revealed comparable results. A 20-week intervention including a low-fat, vegan diet, vitamin B12 supplementation, and weekly support classes for following the prescribed diet lead to significant improvements in individuals with type 2 diabetes and painful diabetic neuropathy. Amongst others, significant improvements in pain were observed in the respective cohort, as measured by the Quality of Life questionnaire and Short Form McGill Pain Questionnaire (Melzack 1975).

Plant-based diets have been shown to exert beneficial health effects with regard to many other chronic conditions including rheumatoid arthritis (Alwarith et al. 2019), heart failure (Kerley 2018, Allen et al. 2019), bronchial asthma (Lindahl et al. 1985, Iikura 2017), diseases of the skin such as psoriasis (Maldonado-Puebla et al. 2019), chronic inflammatory bowel disease (Chiba et al. 2019) such as Crohn's disease (Stewart and Amanda 2018, Sandefur et al. 2019) and retinopathy (Kempner et al. 1958, McGoey-Smith et al. 2019).

The number of studies on vegan and vegetarian diets is continuously rising (Medawar et al. 2019). Their favourable health effects are emphasized in more and more clinical trials and case reports. Ultimately, this development may translate into a new perception of chronic conditions. Chronic diseases, which were once thought to be irreversible and progressive, can actually be stopped and reversed with proper diet. This fundamental shift from managing towards healing has nutrition as the key driver.

Ethical aspects

Such a redefined perception of chronic conditions will inevitably raise a wide range of ethical concerns. Perhaps our current understanding of chronic illness is outdated and morally reprehensible. Physicians may be obligated to recommend a plant-based diet to every single patient suffering from chronic conditions. Finally, other socioecological and economic factors play a role in the process of chronic disease that needs to be evaluated. Considering the current evidence for the effectiveness of plant-based diets, definitions of chronic illness appear to be inadequate and outdated. Remission of clinical symptoms and disease reversal after adopting a plant-based diet have been frequently described.

As a corollary, physicians must consider redefining their understanding of chronic disease. If a cure exists for many pathologies, there are few reasons to still treat just the symptoms. Heart disease is maybe the most impressive example. Instead of prescribing analgesics and nitro-glycerine spray, doctors ought to tackle the root cause of angina. Physicians should dare to routinely prescribe plant-based diets in the same way we prescribe anti-platelet agents or nitrates. The latter is of paramount importance considering the concept of beneficence. This principle requires physicians to prevent and remove harmful conditions from patients (Munyaradzi 2012) and describes the moral obligation to act for the benefit of others (Jahn 2011). Hereby, plant-based nutrition could be a powerful tool and help physicians to prevent harm from occurring to others, e.g. by exposing them to an unhealthy, atherosclerosis-inducing diet.

Medicine does not stand still – it evolves continuously (Snyder 2012). The same should apply to physicians. The ethical principle of utility implies that physician's actions should yield good results, achieving maximum benefits for patients while not wasting precious resources (Nandi 2000). Hence, it is their responsibility and obligation towards their patients to offer evidence-based treatment options. The utilitarian approach asks for medical decisions that allow for the greatest amount of benefits obtained for the largest number of individuals (Mandal *et al.* 2016). For that reason, physicians are obliged to speak out the inconvenient truth. Physicians may no longer ignore the interconnection between nutrition and health. It is time to prescribe healthy diets because medications are by no means a substitute for a dietary intervention (Barnard 2013).

Reducing medication also plays an important role when it comes to the law of therapeutic parsimony (Kalra *et al.* 2016). In place of multiple therapeutic interventions, minimal ones should be used, as long as this can achieve equivalent therapeutic outcomes. If this can be done with a plant-based diet, exposing patients to polypharmacy and its side effects is not only unnecessary, but also potentially harmful. Revisiting the concept of parsimony is also crucial when it comes to a discussion about the economic impact of chronic diseases such as diabetes (Kalra and Saboo 2018). Finally, the major goal must be to get data out to the public where it can actually fundamentally change lives – creating not only longer but also healthier ones (Williams 2017)

Informed consent

The most immediate consequence of this data is that physicians should recommend a plant-based diet to every patient, especially to those who suffer from a chronic condition such as coronary artery disease. It is a valid and evidence-based tool that can reverse conditions that would otherwise slowly progress. Even if a physician is not following a plant-based diet on her own, she should recommend it. The reasons behind this are simple: it is the only diet that has been shown to reverse coronary artery disease (Greger 2015) and because patients should not be denied such knowledge.

Patients have the right to information, which implies that all available treatment options are set forth and clarified. This includes a realistic description of a plant-based diet, including all its benefits and possible challenges, which a patient may experience when changing his nutritional habits. This is an important prerequisite when it comes to the ethical principle of respect for autonomy. The latter refers to the right of self-determination, or that patients have the right to choose what is best for them (French 2006). To allow for autonomy, it is essential to have the necessary information and understanding on which to base a decision. Telling patients the truth by presenting all available treatment options, including fundamental lifestyle changes, is a moral obligation that is derived from the application of respect for autonomy (Jahn 2011).

Of note, autonomy could be diminished by a physician's failure to provide adequate information on which to base a decision. Unfortunately, many physicians lack respect for nutrition as a science and consider fundamental dietary changes unrealistic.

In this context, physicians often stress that a plant-based diet is not for everyone. Some go even further and argue that a plant-based diet is only suitable for a small minority of patients blessed with an iron will and considerable perseverance. The latter, however, is generally questionable. While it is true that not every individual is a candidate to make fundamental changes, one may not predict which patients may adopt a plant-based diet and which patients will not (Klaper 2019). This area warrants further investigation and reliable predictors have not been identified yet. Therefore, it must be tried in clinical practice.

Too often, however, physicians maintain that they have been insufficiently trained in the field of nutrition and lack the time to offer nutrition counselling (Ha 2019). In fact, many physicians do indeed possess insufficient knowledge about nutrition and seem to have an unsatisfactory background to counsel patients on lifestyle (Kris-Etherton *et al.* 2015, Storz 2019). Studies revealed a significant deficiency of nutrition education and practice among internal medicine residents (Vetter *et al.* 2008) and even cardiovascular specialists (Devries *et al.* 2017).

In medicine, however, similar to law, ignorance is no defence. It does not protect against punishment. The World Medical Association's International Code of Medical Ethics leaves no room for interpretation here (World Medical Association 2019), stating, 'Whenever an examination or treatment is beyond the physician's capacity, he/she should consult with or refer to another physician who has the necessary ability.' Therefore, a physician that recognizes the interconnection between health and nutrition can simply refer a patient to a specialist colleague or dietician firm in plant-based nutrition. The latter may not be interpreted as a sign of weakness, but rather as an important effort to provide holistic care.

Physicians should take every available opportunity to incorporate a discussion about nutrition in their daily work. Despite an unfavourable framework including omnipresent time pressure and missing economic incentives to support motivated physicians in plant-based diet counselling (Storz 2019), physicians should keep the bigger picture in mind. Hereby, several landmark papers offer significant practical support and assistance for physicians interested in implementing nutritional advise in daily clinical care (Trapp *et al.* 2010, Hever 2016, Hever and Cronise 2017).

Patients have the right to be told the truth and a plant-based diet should be part of every patient-doctor dialogue. Not mentioning this powerful tool is an act of withholding crucial information.

Socio-ethical implementations

Another important aspect of recommending plant-based diets is the physician's role in society and her responsibility to meet society's health care needs (Brett 2012). According to Lockwood (2004), physicians must serve the community – an important premise that can be traced to the Hippocratic Oath, in which physicians pledge to 'keep [patients] from harm and injustice.' This exhortation to protect society is of uttermost importance, since unhealthy eating habits affect not only a single patient but usually the entire family (Barnard 2013). When parents eat poorly they serve as a negative role model for their own children. Thus, prevalent chronic conditions such as cardiovascular disorders and obesity, spread around a family, like a 'foodborne illness' (Barnard 2013). Maintaining a high level of suspicion of meat-based diets and embarking on constructive discussions about nutrition is therefore a form of fulfilling one's responsibilities and societal obligations. The latter is also in accordance with the World Medical Association's International Code of Medical Ethics, which requires physicians to 'recognize his/her important role in educating the public'.

Offering plant-based options on a regular basis and incorporating them in routine patient care may also be of great interest for hospitals and other healthcare facilities that aim to engage in corporate social responsibility (CSR). The latter has long been a focus of attention (Liu *et al.* 2016) and refers to business operations that involve initiatives benefiting society (Lee *et al.* 2019). While a business' CSR activities can encompass a variety of strategies, implementing greener business operations and environmental efforts is nowadays a common concept (Lee *et al.* 2019). As a corollary, including greener plant-based options in a company's CSR strategy is a powerful tool, since hardly any other CSR measure has a more positive impact than expanding the range of vegan products offered (Albert Schweitzer Foundation 2019). Such an approach might benefit both environmental and human health and could help hospitals to meet their obligation and social responsibilities, e.g. by reducing environmental damage and by protecting animal interests (Brandã *et al.* 2013). Ultimately, CSR activities grow in significance and according to Droppert and Bennett (2015), the global health community would be well-advised to devote itself more to engage in this important practice.

Economic aspects

Currently more than 85% of health care costs are attributable to chronic health conditions in the United States (Beckman 2019, Chapel *et al.* 2017). Drug costs and hospitalizations (Raghupathi and Raghupathi 2018), which are often the consequence of undesired medication side effects, strongly contribute to this number. The price of many medications, such as insulin, continues to rise (Cefalu *et al.* 2018). Out-of-pocket expenses for patients are growing, as well (Patel *et al.* 2018). Consequently, there is a financial incentive to reduce medications. Medicine should be affordable and physicians shall 'strive to use health care resources in the best way to benefit patients and their community' (World Medical Association 2019). Plant-based diets may help to tackle this issue since they have been frequently associated with reduced medication needs (Tuso *et al.* 2013, Hever 2016, Viguiliouk *et al.* 2019) and may therefore help to curb the financial burden from chronic conditions. Beyond this, minimizing medications is good clinical practice and plant-based nutrition may therefore move this concept forward.

According to calculations by Schepers and Annemanns (2018), a wider implementation of plant-based eating would lead to large net economic gains for society. If approximately 10% of the total population in the United Kingdom commit to a high adherence of the Mediterranean diet, societal savings over 20 years are estimated at £7.53 billion. These savings could not only lead to increased financial stability, but also allow for a reallocation of resources given the fact that diets low in meat are associated with better health outcomes. Hereby, it must also be taken into account that a Mediterranean diet usually includes high amounts of olive oil and a moderate intake of fish and poultry (Estruch *et al.* 2018). While according to Ornish (2013) a Mediterranean diet is better than what most people are consuming, a low-fat plant-based diet is even more beneficial. Therefore, even higher benefits and savings are to be expected.

Ultimately, a new data set from the Tzu Chi Vegetarian Study revealed that following a vegetarian diet drastically reduces health care expenses when compared to consuming a diet containing meat (Lin *et al.* 2019). In this study cohort, vegetarians had a 15 percent lower total medical expenditure than persons that consumed meat, fish, and seafood more than once per month.

Ecological aspects

Finally, there are environmental aspects that warrant detailed consideration. The authors of a recently published editorial pointed out that in 2018, the scientific proof for human-induced climate change 'exceeded the gold standard' – the so called '5 Sigma' threshold (Murray *et al.* 2019). This measure is equivalent to a randomized control trial with a p-value of .0000003. Climate change is happening now and the current food system, including its immense dairy and meat production, is a key contributor (Springmann *et al.* 2018). A diet that focuses on animal product consumption, with the accompanying deforestation required to produce grains fed to cattle, is most unsustainable (Plant-Based Nutrition Movement 2019). Therefore, a radical change towards more plant-based diets is critical for avoiding catastrophic environmental damage (Cleveland and Gee 2017). Tackling animal product consumption is crucial in terms of planetary health (Fresán and Sabaté 2019) and animal welfare. Large-scale livestock farming is one of the most significant contributors to environmental problems (Ilea 2009) and raises many ethical concerns.

It is now widely accepted that preventive care has a significantly lower carbon emission than surgical interventions and procedures. The operating theatre is most likely the most resource-intensive part of an hospital (Thiel *et al.* 2015) The production of disposable materials and single-use surgical devices as well as the energy used for air conditioning, heating and ventilation could be drastically reduced by primary prevention. A care strategy primarily focusing on prevention and building on a nutrition-first approach (Ha 2019) is not only better for patients but also for the planet. Such a concept would also achieve the so-called triple bottom line (Slapper and Hall 2011), including sustainability, good health and ultimately financial savings by reducing per capita cost (Wolf 2013).

Conclusion

Plant-based diets have an enormous potential to improve healthcare and to allow for more sustainable medicine. In a recently published review, Fresán and Sabaté emphasized the alignment of health and environmental outcomes for vegetarian diets (2019). Tackling animal product consumption and the intake of saturated fat is consequently not only beneficial with regard to many chronic conditions, but also in terms of planetary health. Protection of the environment is a fundamental responsibility of physicians because they are in a unique position knowing about the interconnection between planetary and human health. Plant-based diets are a powerful tool – not using and advocating for them is not only unethical, but harms patients and the planet alike.

Once plant-based diets receive increased attention and enjoy higher acceptance in the medical community, they will find their way into mainstream medicine. Hereby, both economic and environmental aspects will be the key drivers, along with the numerous health benefits associated with a plant-based diet. This promising scenario and the continuously increasing body of evidence emphasizing the merits of plant-based nutrition will also affect our perception of chronic disease and chronic conditions.

The reservation must be made, however, that the road ahead is long and stony. Plant-based nutrition has not yet been adopted in standard treatment practices by mainstream medicine (Sterling and Bowen 2019) and physicians that follow the 'nutrition-first' approach often encounter considerable resistance (Ha 2019). Despite the meticulous work of renowned experts in the field and the continuously growing body of evidence, the latest findings in this area have not found their way into US national dietetic guidelines (Storz 2019).

Despite these limitations, the plant-based movement could sooner or later redefine our current understanding and perception of chronic conditions. Although a tectonic shift from managing towards curing may raise a number of ethical questions, it will, above all, give new hope and confidence to affected patients, their families and loves ones, while also satisfying numerous ethical demands of informed consent, social and economic wellbeing, and planetary sustainability.

Disclosure statement

No potential conflict of interest was reported by the author(s).

ORCID

Maximilian Andreas Storz http://orcid.org/0000-0003-3277-0301

References

Albert Schweitzer Foundation, 2019. Vegan and meat reduction projects with companies. Available from: https://albertschweitzerfoundation.org/campaigns/vegan-projects-companies. [Accessed 12 March 2020].
Alexander, S., et al., 2017. A plant-based diet and hypertension. *Journal of geriatric cardiology: JGC*, 14 (5), 327–330.
Allen, K.E., Gumber, D. and Ostfeld, R.J., 2019. Heart failure and a plant-based diet. A case-report and literature review. *Frontiers in nutrition*, 6, 82.

Alwarith, J., *et al.*, 2019. Nutrition interventions in rheumatoid arthritis: The potential use of plant-based diets. A review. *Frontiers in nutrition*, 6, 141.

Barnard, N.D., 2007. *Dr. Neal Barnard's program for reversing diabetes*. New York: Rodale.

———., 2013. The physician's role in nutrition-related disorders: from Bystander to Leader. *AMA journal of ethics*, 15 (4), 367–372.

Beckman, K., 2019. A new approach for lifestyle medicine payment. *American journal of lifestyle medicine*, 13 (1), 36–39.

Bell, M.F., *et al.*, 2016. Chronic illness and developmental vulnerability at school entry. *Pediatrics*, 137 (5), doi:10.1542/peds.2015-2475.

Bernell, S. and Howard, S.W., 2016. Use your words carefully: what is a chronic disease? *Frontiers in public health*, 4. doi:10.3389/fpubh.2016.00159.

Boden, W.E., *et al.*, 2007. Optimal medical therapy with or without PCI for stable coronary disease. *The New England journal of medicine*, 356 (15), 1503–1516.

Bodenheimer, T., Chen, E., and Bennett, H.D., 2009. Confronting the growing burden of chronic disease: can the U.S. health care Workforce do the job? *Health affairs*, 28 (1), 64–74.

Bommer, C., *et al.*, 2018. Global economic burden of diabetes in adults: projections from 2015 to 2030. *Diabetes care*, 41 (5), 963–970.

Brandão, C., *et al.*, 2013. Social responsibility: a new paradigm of hospital governance? *Health care analysis*, 21 (4), 390–402.

Brett, A.S., 2012. Physicians have a responsibility to meet the health care needs of society. *The journal of law, medicine & ethics: a journal of the American society of law, medicine & ethics*, 40 (3), 526–531.

British Dietetic Association, 2020. Food Fact Sheet: Plant-based diet. Available from: https://www.bda.uk.com/resource/plant-based-diet.html [Accessed 12 March 2020].

Bunner, A.E., *et al.*, 2015. A dietary intervention for chronic diabetic neuropathy pain: a randomized controlled pilot study. *Nutrition & diabetes*, 5 (5), e158.

Cefalu, W.T., *et al.*, 2018. Insulin access and affordability working group: conclusions and recommendations. *Diabetes care*, 41 (6), 1299–1311.

Chapel, J.M., *et al.*, 2017. Prevalence and medical costs of chronic diseases among adult medicaid beneficiaries. *American journal of preventive medicine*, 53 (6 Suppl 2), S143–S154.

Chiba, M., Ishii, H. and Komatsu, M., 2019. Recommendation of plant-based diets for inflammatory bowel disease. *Translational pediatrics*, 8 (1), 23–27.

Cleveland, D.A. and Gee, Q., 2017. Chapter 9 – plant-based diets for mitigating climate change. In: F. Mariotti, ed. *Vegetarian and plant-based diets in health and disease prevention*. Academic Press, 135–156.

Coulston, A.M., 1999. The role of dietary fats in plant-based diets. *The American journal of clinical nutrition*, 70 (3), 512s–515s.

Crane, M.G. and Sample, C., 1994. Regression of diabetic neuropathy with total vegetarian (vegan) diet. *Journal of nutritional medicine*, 4 (4), 431–439.

Davis, B.C., *et al.*, 2019. An intensive lifestyle intervention to treat type 2 diabetes in the Republic of the Marshall Islands: protocol for a randomized controlled trial. *Frontiers in nutrition*, 6, doi:10.3389/fnut.2019.00079.

de Lorgeril, M., *et al.*, 1999. Mediterranean diet, traditional risk factors, and the rate of cardiovascular complications after myocardial infarction: final report of the Lyon diet heart study. *Circulation*, 99 (6), 779–785.

Devries, S., *et al.*, 2017. A deficiency of nutrition education and practice in cardiology. *The American journal of medicine*, 130 (11), 1298–1305.

Droppert, H. and Bennett, S., 2015. Corporate social responsibility in global health: an exploratory study of multinational pharmaceutical firms. *Globalization and health*, 11 (1), 15. doi:10.1186/s12992-015-0100-5.

Esselstyn, C.B., *et al.*, 2014. A way to reverse CAD? *The journal of family practice*, 63 (7), 356–364b.

Esselstyn, C.B., 2017. A plant-based diet and coronary artery disease: a mandate for effective therapy. *Journal of geriatric cardiology : JGC*, 14 (5), 317–320.

Estruch, R., *et al.*, 2018. Primary prevention of cardiovascular disease with a mediterranean diet supplemented with extra-virgin olive oil or nuts. *New England journal of medicine*, 378 (25), e34.

Feldman, E.L., *et al.*, 2019. Diabetic neuropathy. *Nature reviews disease primers*, 5 (1), 1–18.

French, J., 2006. Introduction to the principles of bioethics. *Canadian journal of medical radiation technology*, 37 (1), 31–36.

Fresán, U. and Sabaté, J., 2019. Vegetarian diets: planetary health and its alignment with human health. *Advances in nutrition*, 10 (Supplement_4), S380–S388.

Greger, M., 2015. Plant-based diets for the prevention and treatment of disabling diseases. *American Journal of lifestyle medicine*, 9 (5), 336–342.

Ha, B., 2019. The power of plants: is a whole-foods, plant-based diet the answer to health, health care, and physician wellness? *The permanente journal*, 23, 3.

Hajat, C. and Stein, E., 2018. The global burden of multiple chronic conditions: a narrative review. *Preventive medicine reports*, 12, 284–293.

Hever, J., 2016. Plant-based diets: a physician's guide. *The permanente journal*, 20 (3), 15–082.

Hever, J. and Cronise, R.J., 2017. Plant-based nutrition for healthcare professionals: implementing diet as a primary modality in the prevention and treatment of chronic disease. *Journal of geriatric cardiology : JGC*, 14 (5), 355–368.

Iikura, M., 2017. 27 – plant-based diets and asthma. In: F. Mariotti, ed. *Vegetarian and plant-based diets in health and disease prevention*. Academic Press, 483–491.

Ilea, R.C., 2009. Intensive livestock farming: global trends, increased environmental concerns, and ethical solutions. *Journal of agricultural and environmental ethics*, 22 (2), 153–167.

Jahn, W.T., 2011. The 4 basic ethical principles that apply to forensic activities are respect for autonomy, beneficence, nonmaleficence, and justice. *Journal of chiropractic medicine*, 10 (3), 225–226.

Juster-Switlyk, K, and Smith, A.G., 2016. Updates in diabetic peripheral neuropathy. F1000Research, 5.

Kahleova, H., Levin, S., and Barnard, N., 2017. Cardio-metabolic benefits of plant-based diets. *Nutrients*, 9 (8), 848. doi:10.3390/nu9080848.

Kalra, S., Gupta, Y., and Sahay, R., 2016. The law of therapeutic parsimony. *Indian journal of endocrinology and metabolism*, 20 (3), 283–284.

Kalra, S. and Saboo, B., 2018. The law of investigative parsimony. *JPMA. The journal of the pakistan medical association*, 68 (5), 817–818.

Kempner, W., Peschel, R.L., and Schlayer, C., 1958. Effect of rice diet on diabetes mellitus associated with vascular disease. *Postgraduate medicine*, 24, 359–371.

Kerley, C.P., 2018. A review of plant-based diets to prevent and treat heart failure. *Cardiac failure review*, 4 (1), 54–61.

Kim, H., et al., 2019. Plant-based diets are associated with a lower risk of incident cardiovascular disease, cardiovascular disease mortality, and all-cause mortality in a general population of middle-aged adults. *Journal of the American heart association*, 8 (16), e012865.

Klaper, M., 2019. What every doctor needs to know about nutrition. conference lecture at VegMed 2019: Europe's biggest scientific conference on plant-based nutrition. 12–13 October, King's College, London, United Kingdom.

Kris-Etherton, P.M., et al., 2015. Nutrition competencies in health professionals' education and training: A new paradigm. *Advances in nutrition*, 6 (1), 83–87.

Lawrence, M.A. and Baker, P.I., 2019. Ultra-processed food and adverse health outcomes. *BMJ*, 365, doi:10.1136/bmj.l2289.

Lee, H., et al., 2019. Public preferences for corporate social responsibility activities in the pharmaceutical industry: Empirical evidence from Korea. *Plos one*, 14 (8), e0221321.

Lin, C.-L., et al., 2019. Vegetarian diets and medical expenditure in Taiwan—a matched cohort study. *Nutrients*, 11 (11), 2688.

Lindahl, O., et al., 1985. Vegan regimen with reduced medication in the treatment of bronchial asthma. *The journal of asthma: official journal of the association for the care of asthma*, 22 (1), 45–55.

Liu, W., et al., 2016. How patients think about social responsibility of public hospitals in China? *BMC health services research*, 16 (1), 371.

Lockwood, A.H., 2004. The physician's role in society: enhancing the health of individuals and the public. *AMA journal of ethics*, 6 (4), 189–190.

Maldonado-Puebla, M., et al., 2019. Efficacy of a plant-based anti-inflammatory diet as monotherapy in psoriasis. *International journal of disease reversal and prevention*, 1 (1), 68–74. https://ijdrp.org/index.php/ijdrp/article/view/15.

Mandal, J., Ponnambath, D.K., and Parija, S.C., 2016. Utilitarian and deontological ethics in medicine. *Tropical parasitology*, 6 (1), 5–7.

Massera, D., et al., 2015. A whole-food plant-based diet reversed angina without medications or procedures. *Case reports in cardiology*, 2015, 978906.

Matthews, D.R. and Matthews, P.C., 2011. Banting memorial lecture 2010^. type 2 diabetes as an 'infectious' disease: is this the Black death of the 21st century? *Diabetic medicine: A journal of the British diabetic association*, 28 (1), 2–9.

McGain, F. and Naylor, C., 2014. Environmental sustainability in hospitals – a systematic review and research agenda. *Journal of health services research & policy*, 19 (4), 245–252.

McGoey-Smith, K., Esselstyn, C. and McGoey-Smith, A., 2019. Reversal of pulmonary hypertension, diabetes, and retinopathy after adoption of a whole food plant-based diet. *International journal of disease reversal and prevention*, 1 (2), 35–44. https://ijdrp.org/index.php/ijdrp/article/view/41.

McMacken, M. and Shah, S., 2017. A plant-based diet for the prevention and treatment of type 2 diabetes. *Journal of geriatric cardiology: JGC*, 14 (5), 342–354.

Medawar, E., et al., 2019. The effects of plant-based diets on the body and the brain: a systematic review. *Translational psychiatry*, 9 (1), 1–17.

Mejia, M.A., et al., 2016. A vegan diet rich in fats of plant origin may reverse coronary artery disease. *The FASEB journal*, 30 (1_supplement), 904.11-904.11.

Melina, V., Craig, W., and Levin, S., 2016. Position of the academy of nutrition and dietetics: vegetarian diets. *Journal of the academy of nutrition and dietetics*, 116 (12), 1970–1980.

Melzack, R., 1975. The McGill pain questionnaire: major properties and scoring methods. *Pain*, 1 (3), 277–299.

Munyaradzi, M., 2012. Critical reflections on the principle of beneficence in biomedicine. *The Pan African medical journal*, 11, 29.

Murray, N., Mack, H.G., and Al-Qureshi, S., 2019. The case for adopting sustainability goals in ophthalmology. *Clinical & experimental ophthalmology*, 47 (7), 837–839.

Myles, I.A., 2014. Fast food fever: reviewing the impacts of the Western diet on immunity. *Nutrition journal*, 13 (1), 61.

Nandi, P.L., 2000. Ethical aspects of clinical practice. *Archives of surgery*, 135 (1), 22–25.

NCD Risk Factor Collaboration, 2016. Worldwide trends in diabetes since 1980: a pooled analysis of 751 population-based studies with 4.4 million participants. *The lancet*, 387 (10027), 1513–1530.

Nowbar Alexandra, N., et al., 2019. Mortality from Ischemic heart disease. *Circulation: cardiovascular quality and outcomes*, 12 (6), e005375.

Ornish, D., et al., 1998. Intensive lifestyle changes for reversal of coronary heart disease. *JAMA*, 280 (23), 2001–2007.

Ornish, D., 2013. Mediterranean diet for primary prevention of cardiovascular disease. *New England journal of medicine*, 369 (7), 675–676. doi:10.1056/NEJMc1306659.

Ostfeld, R.J., 2017. Definition of a plant-based diet and overview of this special issue. *Journal of geriatric cardiology: JGC*, 14 (5), 315.

Pan, W., et al., 2019. Prognostic value of HbA1c for in-hospital and short-term mortality in patients with acute coronary syndrome: a systematic review and meta-analysis. *Cardiovascular diabetology*, 18 (1), 169.

Patel, M.R., et al., 2018. Improving the affordability of prescription medications for people with chronic Respiratory disease. An official American Thoracic Society Policy Statement. *American Journal of respiratory and critical care medicine*, 198 (11), 1367-1374.

Patelakis, E., et al., 2019. Prevalence of vegetarian diet among children and adolescents in Germany. results from EsKiMo II. *Ernahrungs umschau*, 66 (5), 85–91. doi:10.4455/eu.2019.018.

Physicians Committee for Responsible Medicine, 2019. Plant-Based Diets [online]. Available from: https://www.pcrm.org/good-nutrition/plant-based-diets [Accessed 8 Dec 2019].

Pichler, P.P., et al., 2019. International comparison of health care carbon footprints. *Environmental research letters*, 14 (6), 064004.

Plant-Based Nutrition Movement, 2019. UN climate change report calls for change to human diet ... to eat less meat [online]. Available from: https://pbnm.org/ [Accessed 8 December 2019].

Radnitz, C., Beezhold, B., and DiMatteo, J., 2015. Investigation of lifestyle choices of individuals following a vegan diet for health and ethical reasons. *Appetite*, 90, 31-36.

Raghupathi, W. and Raghupathi, V., 2018. An empirical study of chronic diseases in the United States: a visual analytics approach to public health. *International journal of environmental research and public health*, 15, 431.

Rico-Campà, A., *et al.*, 2019. Association between consumption of ultra-processed foods and all cause mortality: SUN prospective cohort study. *BMJ (clinical research ed.)*, 365, l1949.

Sandefur, K., *et al.*, 2019. Crohn's disease remission with a plant-based diet: a case Report. *Nutrients*, 11, 1385.

Satija, A., *et al.*, 2016. Plant-based dietary patterns and incidence of type 2 diabetes in US men and women: results from three prospective cohort studies. *PLos medicine*, 13 (6), e1002039.

——., 2017. Healthful and unhealthful plant-based diets and the risk of coronary heart disease in U.S. adults. *Journal of the American college of cardiology*, 70 (4), 411-422.

Satija, A. and Hu, F.B., 2018. Plant-based diets and cardiovascular health. *Trends in cardiovascular medicine*, 28 (7), 437-441.

Schepers, J. and Annemans, L., 2018. The potential health and economic effects of plant-based food patterns in Belgium and the United Kingdom. *Nutrition*, 48, 24-32.

Sherwani, S.I., *et al.*, 2016. Significance of HbA1c test in diagnosis and prognosis of diabetic patients. *Biomarker insights*, 11, 95-104.

Slapper, T.F. and Hall, T.J., 2011. The triple bottom line: what is it and how does it work? *Indiana business review*, 86 (1), 4-8.

Snyder, L., 2012. American college of physicians ethics manual: sixth edition. *Annals of internal medicine*, 156 (1_Part_2), 73.

Somrongthong, R., *et al.*, 2016. The influence of chronic illness and lifestyle behaviors on quality of life among older Thais. *Biomed research international*, 2016, 2525941.

Springmann, M., *et al.*, 2018. Options for keeping the food system within environmental limits. *Nature*, 562 (7728), 519-525.

Sterling, S.R. and Bowen, S.-A., 2019. The potential for plant-based diets to promote health among blacks living in the United States. *Nutrients*, 11 (12), 2915.

Stewart, D.R. and Amanda, J.S., 2018. Crohn's disease prevention and treatment with a plant-based diet. *Adv res gastroentero hepatol*, 9 (1), 555753. doi:10.19080/ARGH.2018.09.555753.

Stewart, J., Manmathan, G., and Wilkinson, P., 2017. Primary prevention of cardiovascular disease: A review of contemporary guidance and literature. *JRSM cardiovascular disease*, 6, 2048004016687211.

Storz, M.A., 2019. Is there a lack of support for whole-food, plant-based diets in the medical community? *The permanente journal*, 23, 18–068.

Tangvoranuntakul, P., *et al.*, 2003. Human uptake and incorporation of an immunogenic nonhuman dietary sialic acid. *Proceedings of the national academy of sciences of the United States of America*, 100 (21), 12045-12050.

Thiel, C.L., *et al.*, 2015. Environmental impacts of surgical procedures: life cycle assessment of hysterectomy in the United States. *Environmental science & technology*, 49 (3), 1779-1786.

Timko, C.A., Hormes, J.M., and Chubski, J., 2012. Will the real vegetarian please stand up? An investigation of dietary restraint and eating disorder symptoms in vegetarians versus non-vegetarians. *Appetite*, 58 (3), 982–990.

Tomson, C., 2015. Reducing the carbon footprint of hospital-based care. *Future hospital journal*, 2 (1), 57-62.

Tonstad, S., *et al.*, 2013. Vegetarian diets and incidence of diabetes in the Adventist health study-2. *Nutrition, metabolism and cardiovascular diseases*, 23 (4), 292-299.

Trapp, C., Barnard, N., and Katcher, H., 2010. A plant-based diet for type 2 diabetes: The Diabetes Educator.

Tuso, P.J., *et al.*, 2013. Nutritional update for physicians: plant-based diets. *The permanente journal*, 17 (2), 61–66.

Vetter, M.L., *et al.*, 2008. What do resident physicians know about nutrition? An evaluation of attitudes, self-perceived proficiency and knowledge. *Journal of the American college of nutrition*, 27 (2), 287-298.

Viguiliouk, E., *et al.*, 2019. Effect of vegetarian dietary patterns on cardiometabolic risk factors in diabetes: A systematic review and meta-analysis of randomized controlled trials. *Clinical nutrition*, 38 (3), 1133–1145.

Warshaw, G., 2006. Introduction: advances and challenges in care of older people with chronic illness. *Generations*, 30 (3), 5–10.

Whittemore, R. and Dixon, J., 2008. Chronic illness: the process of integration. *Journal of clinical nursing*, 17 (0), 177–187.

Williams, K.A., 2017. Introduction to the 'A plant-based diet and cardiovascular disease' special issue. *Journal of geriatric cardiology: JGC*, 14 (5), 316.

Wolf, J., 2013. The triple aim and the triple Bottom Line. Available from: http://healthierhospitals.org/media-center/spark-blog/triple-aim-and-triple-bottom-line [Accessed 13 Mar 2020].

World Medical Association, 2019. International Code of Medical Ethics [online]. Available from: https://www.wma.net/policies-post/wma-international-code-of-medical-ethics/.

Yokoyama, Y., *et al.*, 2014. Vegetarian diets and blood pressure: a meta-analysis. *JAMA internal medicine*, 174 (4), 577–587.

———., 2014. Vegetarian diets and glycemic control in diabetes: a systematic review and meta-analysis. *Cardiovascular diagnosis and therapy*, 4 (5), 373–382.

Zinöcker, M.K. and Lindseth, I.A., 2018. The western diet–microbiome-host Interaction and Its role in metabolic disease. *Nutrients*, 10 (3), 365.

Going Green: Decreasing Medical Waste in a Paediatric Intensive Care Unit in the United States

Zelda J. Ghersin

Michael R. Flaherty

Phoebe Yager

Brian M. Cummings

The healthcare industry generates significant waste and carbon emissions that negatively impact the environment. Intensive care units (ICU) are a major contributor to the production of waste, due to patient complexity and needs requiring extensive equipment, cleaning practices and pre-emptive supplies. To quantify the extent of the problem, health care professionals collected all unused medical supplies destined to be discarded over three one-week periods in a paediatric intensive care unit, weighed the items, and created an inventory. This article argues for greener hospital standards and provides a specific example of a project framework to reduce disposable waste with the hope that others can embark on similar initiatives for a more ethical and sustainable future for hospitals. Healthcare facilities must not just meet short-sighted safety standards of the now. In order to be a virtuous organization, one must consider all implications of daily decisions, including disposable supplies and cleaning.

Introduction

According to the Lancet Commission on pollution and health, 'pollution is the largest environmental cause of disease and premature death in the world today.' While the effects of pollution on health are mostly seen in developing countries where children, the poor, and the sick are disproportionately affected, in high-income countries pollution-related disease is 'responsible for 1.7% of annual health spending' (Landrigan et al. 2015). Pollution related health issues are not only a problem of rapidly industrializing nations; they are linked to many diseases in developed countries such as the United States.

The burning of fossil fuel produces greenhouse gases that contribute to pollution and drive global warming. The most abundant greenhouse gas (GHG) is carbon dioxide (CO_2). The use and disposal of resources contribute to pollution by exacerbating GHG emissions, such as CO_2, which are linked to a multitude of health issues. Ambient air pollution has significant effects on health, with increased rates of heart attacks, pulmonary disease and cancer all linked to pollution (Wang et al. 2015, Kurt et al. 2016). Furthermore, certain neurocognitive disorders such as autism, attention deficit disorder and decreased cognitive function are also linked to increased pollution (Weuve 2012, Volk et al. 2013, Perera et al. 2014). In paediatrics, asthma exacerbation is one of the most common indications for admission to the intensive care unit and is linked to air pollution. In 10 cities in Europe, living alongside a busy road in urban areas was associated with acute asthma exacerbations that were otherwise preventable (Perez et al. 2013).

A recent report by the US Environmental Protection Agency found that in 2018, US greenhouse gas totalled 6677.8 million metric tons of carbon dioxide equivalents (mmtCO2eq) and was responsible for 15% of total global emissions (2020). While the total amount of US GHG production has decreased over the past 10 years, the healthcare system continues to be a major contributor to overall GHG production.

This article aims to explore how wasteful practices have become engrained in the healthcare industry culture and the ethical imperative to address it. The article also details efforts to create a 'greener' future in the paediatric intensive care unit (PICU) of Massachusetts General Hospital for Children, Boston as a model for other inpatient units embarking on similar initiatives. As climate activist Greta Thunberg (2019) once remarked, the eyes of all future generations are upon us. As future generations watch, we must identify and implement strategies to reduce the production of medical waste while also maximizing opportunities to reuse and recycle.

The culture of waste in healthcare

The healthcare industry generates significant waste and carbon emissions that negatively impact the environment. Carbon emissions are not in everyday consciousness since they are not tangible or visible on a daily basis. Excessive waste has therefore become deeply-rooted in US healthcare culture since the effects of processing that waste are not overtly seen. A recent study attributed as much as 25% of all US healthcare spending as wasteful, with an accumulated debt between $760 and 935 billion dollars (Shrank *et al.* 2019). This economic waste is due to unnecessary testing, overtreatment, inappropriate pricing, as well as care coordination and administrative failures. Inefficient spending practices are mirrored in environmentally wasteful practices that are stimulated by an abundance of easily accessible supplies that are sparsely regulated. In the hospital setting, this is mostly seen in operating rooms and labour and delivery units, as they are the largest contributors to hospital waste (Woods *et al.* 2015).

The generation and processing of medical waste in the US healthcare system have not been sufficiently studied until recently. Practice Greenhealth (2019), an organization that provides environmentally sustainable solutions for the healthcare industry, reports each hospital bed contributes 11 kg/bed/day and that hospitals create 5.9 million tons of waste annually. Utilizing these estimates, a hospital with 1000 beds may generate 11,300 kg of waste per day. To put this into perspective, that is two full dumptrucks of garbage each day for a large size hospital.

While the sheer weight of medical waste alone is impressive, cradle-to-grave life cycle analysis (LCA) of different medical supplies quantify each product's environmental impact. These types of analysis follow a product from its processing and development to its disposal to analyse the total environmental impact over its lifetime. The use of LCAs allows us to consciously purchase supplies that have a less environmental impact. In a study evaluating the impact of four different surgical procedures, it was found that the major sources of environmental emissions included the production of disposable materials and single-use surgical devices (Thiel *et al.* 2015). Similarly, an LCA of all the equipment used in the birth of a baby (both vaginal and caesarean section) concluded that the production and disposal of the single-use custom packs (containing surgical instrumentation) had one of the largest environmental impacts of the entire birthing process (Campion *et al.* 2012). As these studies suggest, the increase in single-use disposable medical supplies has not only amplified the production of frank waste, but may also significantly contribute to total GHG emissions in the healthcare sector.

The culture of waste in intensive care units

While the ICU is not the main contributor to wasteful practices in the inpatient setting, it does add a significant amount of waste, mostly due to the procedures and advanced equipment used to support life. When taking care of critically ill patients in the ICU, the emergency department, or an operating room, all decision-making processes err on the side of caution. Nurses, respiratory therapists and physicians anticipate crisis in an effort to be prepared should the worst-case scenario occur. This judicious preparation is intended to be in the best interest of the patient, yet it also contributes to wasteful practices.

This is especially true in the PICU where critically ill and injured children and their families judiciously watch every flurry of action. Beyond observing bedside rounds and nurses constantly adjusting monitors and titrating medication pumps, children watch every move of their caregivers – even when we think they are too sick to notice. They watch and learn as we discard countless syringes, tubings, plastic encasings, bedpans and complex medical apparatuses. They watch as we open a 10 French nasogastric tube, only to realize that we needed an 8 French and thoughtlessly toss it out. They watch as the cleaning staff remove three full garbage bins of waste per shift, a mixture of both soiled and unused products. These everyday experiences highlight an enormous problem facing healthcare and send an unintended message to our youth regarding acceptable wasteful behaviours and planet stewardship.

A commonly observed scenario seen in the ICU occurs when nurses and respiratory therapists prepare for a patient in respiratory distress. By the bedside they open and organize all supplies required for placement of a breathing tube, if needed. Intubation blades, handles, endotracheal tubes, stylets, oropharyngeal airways, laryngeal mask airways and resuscitator bags with masks are only a handful of the items they may open from sterilized packages. Yet, most patients respond well to less invasive therapies and never require a breathing tube, in which case all of these supplies are discarded.

Nurses, who spend the most time by the patient's bedside, are taught that having everything opened and ready to use will prepare the entire medical team should the patient deteriorate. They do not want to feel ill-equipped when doctors enter the room in an emergency situation. In addition to this rationale, preparedness is also attributed to professionalism – if you are not prepared you may have failed the patient. Despite this, most units have airway and code carts where equipment is readily available should an emergency ensue. There remains a fine balance between appropriate preparation to guarantee the safe care of a critically ill patient and excessive preparation of medical supplies that often go unused. In a high acuity environment, the scales are generally tipped in favour of overpreparation and excessive caution, even when alternative pathways exist.

A report from the American Psychological Association Taskforce (2009) on the interface between psychology and global climate change identified several reasons why hospital staff may not engage in practices that are environmentally friendly. Among these reasons are beliefs that individual action is not enough, someone higher up is dealing with the problem, or the feeling of being overwhelmed with the crisis and being unsure of how to help. For instance, in our PICU, it is a common notion that excessive waste is so widespread that any individual attempt to decrease the amount of waste produced by the bedside is insignificant. Compared to the waste produced in the operating room, cafeteria, or the pharmacy, what is one more wasted endotracheal tube, stylet or oxygen mask? The fallacy that individual action will not create a measurable difference hardens this culture of indifference. This lends itself to a culture where no one assumes the burden of responsibility. However, as Margaret Mead's famous quote reads 'never doubt that a small group of thoughtful, committed citizens can change the world; indeed, it's the only thing that ever has' (Lutkehaus 2008).

The concept of diffusion of responsibility – in particular – has also been suggested to play a role in the culture of indifference towards environmental sustainability in health care organizations (Topf 2005). Individuals may incorrectly assume that other colleagues or departments are taking control of waste management, or that there are hospital-wide sustainability programmes in place. In other words, the responsibility should fall on the upper echelon of hospital administration to develop interventions to decrease the hospital's environmental impact rather than the individual.

The Joint Commission on Accreditation of Healthcare Organizations

Indeed, in an effort to meet national standards such as those stipulated by the Joint Commission on Accreditation of Healthcare Organizations (JAHCO), hospitals have adopted certain practices to minimize hospital-associated morbidity and mortality. This, of course, has high ethical validity – we must avoid harming our patients, or at a minimum do everything we know to prevent harm. One of the main targets of JAHCO is infection control.

While initially focused on sterilization techniques, infection control has evolved to accommodate outbreaks of disease. The *LA Times* cited several deaths that were linked to a superbug thought to be from contaminated medical scopes (Terhune 2015). Since then, the U.S. Food and Drug Administration has released a recommendation to transition to the use of duodenoscopes that have disposable parts (2019). This is an example of hospitals moving towards disposable medical supplies in order to prevent these hospital-acquired and communicable infections. Gowns, intubation equipment, and surgical kits that were once reusable after sterilization are now discarded after a single-use. In addition, the abundance of these supplies in stock allows providers to carelessly toss away equipment even if it was never used on a patient.

While it has been argued that the energy required to clean and sterilize reusable medical equipment may have a larger environmental burden than the disposal of single-use devices, recent life cycle analysis (LCA) of common medical supplies suggests otherwise. In a study comparing single-use versus reusable medical supplies, several medical products, such as scissors and laryngeal mask airways, were found to have lower life-cycle greenhouse gases when used as a reusable as opposed to a single-use disposable (Unger *et al.* 2016). Scissors exhibited the highest emissions of CO_2 when used as a stainless-steel single-use disposable. Furthermore, disposable medical supplies also need to be sterilized before being packaged. These sterilization procedures require large amounts of water, energy, and chemical disinfectants that also impact their cradle-to-grave life cycle. Until more LCAs are conducted on common medical equipment the true environmental burden of this shift towards single-use supplies will remain unknown.

Another infection control measure with a high environmental burden is the handling of medical supplies in contact precaution rooms. Contact isolation precautions are used for infections that are spread by touching the infected patient or items in their room. This requires all hospital staff to wear gowns to cover their clothing and gloves when entering the patient's room. The purpose of these precautions is to prevent the spread of infection to other patients. Strict guidelines set by infection control committees, following standards from JAHCO, require most of the contents in a contact precaution room to be discarded when the patient is discharged. While many supplies are stored securely away in medical carts and may never have been in contact with a patient or their providers, at the time of discharge they are often discarded for fear of possible contamination. Once a screening swab or viral panel is sent, the patient is placed in contact isolation until the results become available. Many times, patients are transferred or discharged with results still pending. These rooms are still considered isolation and all their contents must be discarded appropriately even when the clinical suspicion of transmittable infection is very low. These supplies are not recycled and end up in landfills, further contributing to the healthcare industry's environmental footprint.

It has been suggested that when more than 40% of hospitalized patients are placed on contact precautions, adherence to these precautions decreases (Dhar et al. 2014). Hospitals should develop strict guidelines that dictate screening panels only for patients with a high clinical suspicion of having disease. This would not only decrease excessive medical testing but also decrease the wasteful practices associated with placing patients in contact isolation.

While the intent of JAHCO is to improve the delivery of healthcare and protect patients from harm, strict regulations that are instituted by hospitals in order to gain accreditation are actually worsening wasteful practices, creating a new source of future patient harm, and perhaps not even meeting its stated intention. In a study that analysed 4400 hospitals in the US, being accredited by an independent organization such as JAHCO did not decrease patient risk of mortality (Lam et al. 2018).

The increased use and production of disposables to protect patients and meet JAHCO standards has the inadvertent effect of causing the US healthcare system to exacerbate its GHG burden. The environmental effects of increased pollution have a direct impact on health. The medical industry is caught in a self-perpetuating cycle. There is a need for increased responsibility of healthcare providers to take a more active role in minimizing carbon footprint while still safely taking care of patients.

On the other hand, a more hardline view taken by some bioethicists is that our culture to save life no matter the cost is not sustainable in the long run. 'Achievements in life expectancy may be associated with an unsustainable use of natural resources and an unsustainable production of wastes' (Dwyer 2009). The extreme measures we take to prolong life have a large environmental cost that, from a bioethical viewpoint, harms society as a whole. There must be a better way forward.

The way forward, quality improvement

Doctors, nurses and ancillary hospital staff must take ownership, start formulating, and put into action interventions that will create a measurable change towards sustainability. The authors embarked on a way to better assess the impact our decisions were having in our local environment and contributing to the short-sightedness of the healthcare industry. In order to tackle the larger issue of waste, we had to start with what we were doing. Here lies the professional and ethical imperative to assess performance, reflect, and constantly improve. Quality improvement provides the framework for ethical everyday practice in an outwardly demanding

ICU world. An example of this approach is the following case study in applied sustainability in a PICU in Boston (US).

Care team
The PICU at Massachusetts General Hospital for Children/Harvard Medical School in Boston Massachusetts is a 14-bed medical/surgical ICU with approximately 1200 admissions per year. The unit is staffed by paediatric residents, emergency medicine residents, paediatric critical care fellows, paediatric critical care attendings (one who has a background in ethics), nurses, and respiratory therapists. Additionally, there are nutritionists, pharmacists, physical and occupational therapists, social workers, child life specialists and medical students that are part of the multidisciplinary team. Thus, we are a unit of interprofessionals dedicated to the higher good of helping children in need. This Boston PICU treats children with life-threatening issues such as sepsis, respiratory failure, trauma, burns and post-operative management. All modern tools are at our disposal. Patients are supported by advanced medical technology including invasive and non-invasive mechanical ventilation, neurologic monitoring, extracorporeal membrane oxygenation (ECMO) and dialysis.

Creation of a Green Team and a shared vision
A busy unit with acutely ill patients is expected to generate a large amount of waste. In order to address some of our wasteful practices a 'Green Team' was created. Like all movements, it started internally and then grew to include a larger group of providers that also voiced their concerns of excessive waste production. The team included physicians at all levels of training, nurses and respiratory therapists. All were concerned about the amount of medical waste produced by our unit on a daily basis. Each member volunteered their time to start an initiative and act as champions of change.

A mission statement for the Green Team was devised to guide the team: 'to develop high impact strategies towards the creation of a zero-carbon emissions model in the PICU.' From that mission and vision, the first tactic was devised – to decrease the amount of medical waste produced daily. This required effective ways to reduce waste production and implement strategies towards reusing and recycling. By striving to be carbon neutral, the Green Team aims to create a sustainable workplace that employees are proud of, with the belief that this will translate to a higher quality of care, enhanced patient experience, and ultimately, a world we can all live in. With motivated staff, this process improvement initiative can be replicated in any hospital in the US or the world. The team followed the quality improvement methodology of developing a problem statement, setting a timeline and charter, obtaining diagnostic data and brainstorming interventions to start improving.

Problem statement and aims
A majority of medical waste in the paediatric intensive care unit (PICU) comes from medical equipment that is brought into a patient's room, and either opened and unused, or never opened but cannot be reused and is thus wasted. This excessive waste increases the unit's carbon footprint and leads to increased resource

acquisition. By developing a standardized approach to minimize excess waste of unused medical materials the team intended to reduce the overall waste consumption of this unit. Furthermore, there is an added financial benefit for the economic longevity of the unit to decrease the amount of medical supplies that are purchased.

Methods
Several meetings were held to define the project's aims, timeline and roadmap. Members of the Green Team, as well as nurse managers, unit attendings and fellows were present at these meetings and acted as advisors for the project. Key partnerships were established, including environmental services and infection control. A significant starting point for diagnostic data was determining which items normally thrown out could be safely collected and stored in a soiled utility closet to quantify. After itemization, they could be discarded through traditional processes. To ensure staff participation beyond the Green Team, traditional change management concepts and communication were used. A short presentation was distributed to all staff members describing our quality improvement initiative. Green Team members took on the role as unit champions to support and motivate their colleagues during collection periods and oversee the proper collection of waste throughout the shift and during patient discharge. For all shifts, at least one Green Team member was identified.

Unused medical waste was defined as opened or unopened medical equipment that is brought into a patient's room and not used. Multiple items were excluded from collection including medications, sharps, opened liquids, soiled items and food. The exclusion of these items were decided based on safety, feasibility and scope of project. During the collection period, bedside nurses in the PICU were asked to place unused medical equipment that they would normally throw into the trash into specialized, marked containers. Each day these containers were weighed. The contents collected were then sorted and inventoried to identify the most commonly wasted items.

To ensure that all staff understood the aim of the diagnostic phase and how it would impact their daily workflow, the initiative was reviewed at the start of each shift at a huddle. During these brief huddles, a member of the Green Team would review the inclusion and exclusion criteria of items that were to be collected, as well as the proper disposal of waste that was deemed unused. Before a patient admission, rooms were stocked as they normally would be. Since the cleaning staff is responsible for the disposal of all waste in the unit, we handed out presentations and reviewed the details of the project with each member during collection days. Since we hypothesized that the majority of unused supplies would be wasted at the time of patient discharge, we asked that both the nurse and a member of the cleaning staff be present at the time of discharge to collect all remaining waste before the room was completely cleaned.

Findings
A total of 76 kg of unused medical waste was collected over a three-week period. The majority of waste was collected at the time of patient transfer or discharge.

Based on medical records, it was estimated that greater than 75% of the waste came from isolation rooms. The most commonly disposed items were endotracheal tubes (150), diapers (104), disposable underpads (47) and flexible suction catheters (42) (see Table 1). Other smaller items discarded in bulk were port protector caps (infection control devices for invasive lines), medical dressings (e.g. sticky clear covers for IVs), syringes and mouth care swabs. The costs were also quantified in US dollars (Vitality Medical 2019). The most expensive items that were discarded were four tracheostomy tubes, 2 of them custom made, which cost between $200 and 500 each, 10 disposable oxygen saturation measurement probes (approx. $40 each), 31 resuscitator bags ($15–31 depending on size) 1 cooling blanket gel pad ($169) and 1 oscillating positive end expiratory pressure therapy system ($89). The vast majority of items collected were unopened. The team also noted that although there should be only one disposable stethoscope per room, multiple stethoscopes (up to three) were found in several patient rooms.

Limitations

There are several limitations to the Boston-based quality improvement initiative. There may be items included in the analysis that were used but discarded in the collection bins. This risk was mitigated by reminding staff that we were in a collection period at the start of each shift and attempting to have both a nurse and cleaning staff present to empty the room at the time of patient discharge. Another limitation is that some nurses have the thoughtful practice of returning items to the clean utility closet that were unused, as long as they were not in an isolation room. We did not encourage those nurses to throw out items they were planning on returning for reuse. Daily staff were reminded to continue with their normal practices and in the presentations, the importance of continuing each individual's typical workflow was stressed. Finally, our unit is medium-sized and other units may feel similar

TABLE 1.
MOST COMMONLY DISPOSED ITEMS.

Item	Amount	Estimated cost per item (USD)
Endotracheal tube	150	$ 2.00
Diaper	104	$ 0.40
Disposable under pad	47	$ 1.16
Flexible suction catheter	42	$ 0.45–0.50
Intubation stylet	39	$ 2.50–5.50
Oral airway	38	$ 0.96–1.00
Rigid suction catheter	36	$ 1.02
Resuscitator Bag + Mask	31	$ 15.96–31.78
Capnometer	29	$ 2.00
Pack of diaper wipes	21	$ 3.36
Feeding tube	20	$ 1.37
PEEP valve	17	$ 3.75

initiatives are out of reach. On the contrary, any unit, despite their size, can create a Green Team. Larger units may even find that they have more intervenable practices towards limiting their environmental footprint.

Possible interventions

The overall reduction of items stocked inside patient rooms may have the largest impact on the amount of unused medical waste produced. This requires a change in culture and practice. Many providers believe that it is their professional duty to have contingency plans for possible emergencies. However, these precautions are already in place – the unit has carts outside of patient rooms with all needed supplies that are designed to be easily accessible in the case of an airway emergency. Although these carts exist and nurses are encouraged to use them, the practice of waste persists because of this engrained professional duty to prepare and anticipate. One way to frame this conundrum is that over-preparation is actually harming future patients from carbon emissions that lead to climate change health hazards.

Moreover, over-preparation does not meet the biomedical principle of justice, since resources are not used appropriately. A justice framework requires that health care professionals use resources wisely and limit over-preparation. Stocking rooms can be phased out and, rather than bringing individual devices to the bedside, providers can place the supply airway cart directly outside the patient's room when needed.

Another intervention using the justice principle involves protecting bedside resuscitator bags, positive end-expiratory pressure (PEEP) valves and oropharyngeal airways inside plastic bags so they can be re-used. The Green Team is currently developing guidelines to limit the amount of supplies stocked in each room. The guidelines will set limits on the number of diapers, suction catheters, end tidal CO_2 detectors, wipes and disposable underpads brought into a room at a given time. A *Waste Limiting Checklist* that reminds staff how to properly stock rooms and care for equipment so it can be reused will motivate staff to limit their waste production. This intervention will have the greatest impact on reducing the large quantity of resources thrown out, follow valid ethical principles, and save our environment.

By setting an example, the PICU Green Team will encourage medical peers to transition towards environmentally conscious purchasing. This project has the potential to enact a cultural change by including environmentally thoughtful resource acquisition, such as purchasing supplies that are recyclable or biodegradable and buying from companies that conduct and share life-cycle-analysis of their supplies. Other ICUs have implemented waste audits that are driven by feedback and incentives (Chapman and Chapman 2011).

There has already been a push towards the creation of 'life cycle inventory databases' which will help guide responsible purchasing (Sherman *et al.* 2019). This can be instituted for the purchasing of medical supplies as well. Finally, any unused medical supplies can be repurposed for simulation-based medical education, and unused equipment can be donated to families and hospitals in low resourced settings.

Conclusion

Hospitals, as an institution, were created with the primary aim of treating the unwell. Yet, the healthcare sector is a major contributor to GHG emissions in many countries. This, ironically, contributes to pollution-related disease that hospitals must treat. Committees such as JAHCO seek to improve the delivery of healthcare by reducing morbidities such as hospital-acquired and transmitted infections. In order to meet these standards and gain accreditation, one of the effects has been the move towards single-use disposable medical supplies and the implementation of hospital-wide policies that exacerbate already wasteful practices. Through newer life-cycle-analysis of different medical supplies, there is empirical evidence on which items have the worst impact on the environment. Yet, until more studies are conducted, it will be up to each individual and unit to establish their own environmentally responsible practices.

To this end, doctors, nurses and ancillary hospital staff must find ways to balance the professional duty to prepare with the professional duty to limit the negative impact practices have on the environment, and to save resources when able. Health care professionals have the responsibility to be stewards of resource consumption and disposal and to act in accordance with the principle of justice towards future generations that will bear the burden of current environmentally harmful practices. The development of a Green Team whose first project was to decrease the amount of unused medical waste produced in a Boston PICU was a call to action.

By sharing this successful project, other inpatient units can be empowered to develop similar initiatives. By encouraging staff to go green, health care professionals can create a more sustainable PICU of which employees are proud. This will translate to improved patient care. In our world, the eyes of future generations watch us at all times. There is an ethical obligation to set an example for them.

Disclosure statement

No potential conflict of interest was reported by the author(s).

References

Campion, N., *et al.*, 2012. Life cycle assessment perspectives on delivering an infant in the US. *Science of the total environment*, 425, 191–198.

Chapman, M., and Chapman, A., 2011. Greening critical care. *Critical care*, 15 (2), 302.

Dhar, S., *et al.*, 2014. Contact precautions more Is not necessarily better. *Infection control & hospital epidemiology*, 35 (3), 213–219.

Dwyer, J., 2009. How to connect bioethics and environmental ethics: health, sustainability, and justice. *Bioethics*, 23 (9), 497–502.

Kurt, O.K., Zhang, J., and Pinkerton, K.E., 2016. Pulmonary health effects of air pollution. *Current opinion in pulmonary medicine*, 22 (2), 138–143.

Lam, M.B., *et al.*, 2018. Association between patient outcomes and accreditation in US hospitals: observational study. *Bmj*, 363:k4011.

Landrigan, P.J., Fuller, R., and Horton, R., 2015. Environmental pollution, health, and development: a Lancet–global alliance on health and pollution – Icahn School of Medicine at Mount Sinai Commission. *The Lancet*, 386 (10002), 1429–1431.

Lutkehaus, N.C., 2008. *Margaret Mead: the making of an American Icon*. Princeton, NJ: Princeton University Press, 261.

Perera, F.P., *et al.*, 2014. Early-life exposure to polycyclic aromatic hydrocarbons and ADHD behavior problems. *PLos ONE*, 9, 11.

Perez, L., *et al.*, 2013. Chronic burden of near-roadway traffic pollution in 10 European cities. *ISEE Conference abstracts*, 2013 (1), 5880.

Practice Greenhealth. 2019. Waste [online]. Available from: https://practicegreenhealth.org/topics/waste [Accessed 9 Dec 2019].

2009. *Psychology and global climate change: addressing a multi-faceted phenomenon and set of challenges*. Report of the American Psychological Association Task Force on the interface between Psychology and Global Climate Change. Available from: https://www.apa.org/science/about/publications/climate-change [Accessed 9 Dec 2019]

Sherman, J.D., Macneill, A., and Thiel, C., 2019. Reducing pollution from the health care industry. *Jama*, 322 (11), 1043.

Shrank, W.H., Rogstad, T.L., and Parekh, N., 2019. Waste in the US health care system. *Jama*, 322 (15), 1501.

Terhune, C. 2015. Superbug linked to 2 deaths at UCLA hospital; 179 potentially exposed. *Los Angeles Times*, 18 February. Available from: https://www.latimes.com/business/la-fi-hospital-infections-20150218-story.html. [Accessed 9 December 2019].

Thiel, C.L., *et al.*, 2015. Environmental impacts of surgical procedures: life cycle assessment of hysterectomy in the United States. *Environmental science & technology*, 49 (3), 1779–1786.

Thunberg, G. 2019. The UN Climate Summit, New York. NBC News. TV. Sept 23.

Topf, M., 2005. Psychological explanations and interventions for indifference to greening hospitals. *Health care management review*, 30 (1), 2–8.

Unger, S.R., *et al.*, 2016. Evaluating quantifiable metrics for hospital green checklists. *Journal of cleaner production*, 127, 134–142.

United States Environmental Protection Agency, 2020. *Inventory of U.S. Greenhouse Gas Emissions and Sink: 1990-2018*. Washington: United States Government.

2019. U.S. Food and Drug Administration Recommendation on Health Care Facilities and Manufacturers begin transitioning to duodenoscopes with disposable components to reduce risk of patient infection.

Vitality Medical. 2019. Available from: https://www.vitalitymedical.com/. [Accessed 2 March 2020].

Volk, H.E., *et al.*, 2013. Traffic-related air pollution, particulate matter, and autism. *JAMA Psychiatry*, 70 (1), 71.

Wang, X., Kindzierski, W. and Kaul, P., 2015. Air pollution and acute myocardial infarction hospital admission in Alberta, Canada: a three-step procedure case-crossover study. *Plos One*, 10 (7).

Weuve, J., 2012. Exposure to particulate air pollution and cognitive decline in older women. *Archives of internal medicine*, 172 (3), 219.

Woods, D.L., *et al.*, 2015. Carbon footprint of robotically-assisted laparoscopy, laparoscopy and laparotomy: a comparison. *The international Journal of medical Robotics and Computer Assisted Surgery*, 11 (4), 406–412.

Index

Annemans, L. 78
anthropogenic climate degradation 43
attention restoration theory (ART) 43
autonomy 35, 36, 76, 77

Barnard, N.D. 74
Bennett, S. 78
biodiversity 24, 33, 34
Boston-based quality improvement initiative 94
Bunner, A.E. 75

cardiovascular disease 69, 70, 72
care team 92
Carroll, L. 58
carte blanche 64
catechism 56, 57
chronic diseases 6, 69–80
chronic illness 69, 70, 75
civil disobedience 62
climate change 15, 16, 32, 33, 36, 39, 41, 42, 46, 56, 57, 62, 64–66
climate crisis 39, 66
climate emergency 4, 6, 55, 63–65
conflicts 15, 16, 18, 24–27, 56, 62, 64
Conly, S. 22
contemporary bioethics 14, 15
culture of waste 87, 88; in healthcare 87–88; in intensive care units 88–91

diabetes 34, 35, 69–71, 73–76
diabetic neuropathy 74–75
disease reversal 70, 72, 73, 75
Droppert, H. 78
dual use dilemma 35

Eckelman, M.J. 46
ecological aspects 79
economic aspects 78–79
ecotherapy 6, 42–45; Markevych's three pathways of 43–44; and veterans 44–45
empirical medicine 31, 32
energy efficiency 48, 49
entropy 33, 34

environmental/environment 4, 5, 14–16, 18, 20, 21, 23, 25, 26, 34, 36, 39, 40, 42, 43, 46, 47, 51; degradation 20, 38, 39, 46; ethics 4–6, 14, 15, 31, 36, 40; exploitation 6, 7; impacts 4, 7, 14–16, 21, 88, 90; protection 14–18, 21, 24, 26, 27; resources 14, 15, 17–20, 23, 24, 26, 27, 40
environmental health 4, 7, 21–23, 25, 50; promotion 22, 23
Esselstyn, C.B. 73
ethical aspects 75–76
ethical codes 58, 61, 66
ethical foundations 48, 56
extinction rebellion 6, 56, 62–64, 66; doctors for 62–63

food system 7, 23, 24, 26
Frumkin, H. 48, 49

General Medical Council (GMC) 6, 56–57, 59, 60, 62–66
global emergency 8
global health ethic 50, 51
Goldberg, T. 51
golden rule 56–58, 61, 62, 65, 66
green health care centres 46, 47
green health centres 6, 50
greenspace 43, 44
Green Team 5, 92, 93, 95, 96
Greger, M. 74

Hajat, C. 69
Hawkins, B. 45
health benefits 41, 42, 45, 80
health care 3–8, 14–19, 21, 38, 39, 42, 46–50, 66; costs 70, 78; facilities 3, 4; professionals 19, 20, 63; providers 6, 7
health centres 45
health effects 42, 43, 75
health promotion 7, 14–18, 21, 24, 26, 27; synergy of 18–21
Hedberg, T. 22
Held, V. 46
Horton, R. 42

human body 5, 31–34, 42, 55, 71
humanity 33, 51
humankind 36, 55, 56
human population 22, 23
human relationship 35, 40

informed consent 76–77, 80
initial secular pledges 59
innovations 16, 17, 35
integrative building design 48, 50

Jennings, Bruce 16

Kahleova, H. 71
Kahneman, D. 57

Leadership in Energy and Environmental Design (LEED) 49
Lockwood, A.H. 77

Markevych, I. 42
medical ethics 40, 45, 47, 59, 77, 78
medical knowledge 48
medical waste 5–7, 87, 88, 92; decreasing 86–96
moral obligations 76
mosquitoes 24, 25, 39
Mumps, Measles and Rubella (MMR) combined immunization 58

national professional regulators 59–61
natural ecosystem 5, 31–36
nature 3, 4, 6, 33, 34, 39–46, 48, 50; mirror 33; therapies 38, 40, 42, 44, 45
non-human environment 38, 39, 42
nurses 32, 88, 89, 91–96
nutrition 23, 72, 75–78
nutrition-first approach 70, 79, 80

observational climate 32–33
Ornish, Dean 72, 79
Osler, Sir William 34
Ostfeld, R.J. 71

paediatric intensive care unit (PICU) 5, 87–89, 92, 93; in United States 86–96
patient autonomy 45
patient care 5, 45, 47, 50
Patz, J. 51
personal health 35–36
pharmaceutical waste 18
physician activism 62
planetary health 4, 35–36, 50, 56, 59, 79, 80
plant-based diets 7, 71–80
plant-based movement 69–80
plant-based nutrition 73, 76–78, 80; and vegan diets 70–72
pollution 39, 43, 47, 87
population health 16–19, 23

possible interventions 95
Potter, Van Rensselaer 8
problem statement 92
procedural accountability 36
public health 6, 14, 38–42, 47–50, 55, 63, 64, 66; campaigns 35; ethics 15, 16

quality improvement 60, 62, 91

radical activists 62, 63
radical examples 21–26
recycle 48, 49, 87
responsibilities 15, 20, 21, 24–27, 35, 36, 41, 42, 76–78, 89
Restorative Commons 38–42, 44, 45, 47, 48, 50, 51
reuse 47–49, 87, 92, 94, 95
Rieder, T.N. 22
right minded professionals 6, 55, 64
Roberts, David 55

Sackett, C.R. 42
Schepers, J. 78
Second Law of Thermodynamics 34
self-determination 76
Semmelweis, Ignaz 32
shared vision 92
Sherman, J. 46
social environments 16
socio-ethical implementations 77–78
solidarity 15, 16
Stein, E. 69
stem cells 34
survival 8
sustainability 6, 38, 39, 45–51, 79, 80, 89–91; in green health care centres 46–47; in traditional health care centres 45–46
sustainable health care 3, 4, 6
Swift, Jonathan 57

Thunberg, G. 87
traditional health care centres 45–46
type 2 diabetes 34, 73–74

unhealthful vegan diets 71
unused medical waste 93, 95, 96

veterans 42, 44, 45

war on terror 44
waste, quantify 49
wasteful practices 87, 88, 91, 92, 96
whistleblowers 55, 63, 65–66; reluctant 55
whistleblowing 62, 65
World Health Organization 14, 24, 32
wound healing 34

Yokoyama, Y. 73, 74

Milton Keynes UK
Ingram Content Group UK Ltd.
UKHW052022050424
440453UK00003B/4